New Trends in Cognitive Ageing and Mild Cognitive Impairment

New Trends in Cognitive Ageing and Mild Cognitive Impairment

Editors

David Facal
Carlos Spuch
Sonia Valladares Rodriguez

MDPI • Basel • Beijing • Wuhan • Barcelona • Belgrade • Manchester • Tokyo • Cluj • Tianjin

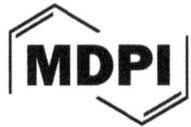

Editors
David Facal
University of Santiago de
Compostela
Spain

Carlos Spuch
Galicia Sur Health Research
Institute
Spain

Sonia Valladares Rodriguez
University of Vigo
Spain

Editorial Office
MDPI
St. Alban-Anlage 66
4052 Basel, Switzerland

This is a reprint of articles from the Special Issue published online in the open access journal *Geriatrics* (ISSN 2308-3417) (available at: https://www.mdpi.com/journal/geriatrics/special_issues/aging_cognitive_2).

For citation purposes, cite each article independently as indicated on the article page online and as indicated below:

LastName, A.A.; LastName, B.B.; LastName, C.C. Article Title. *Journal Name* **Year**, *Volume Number*, Page Range.

ISBN 978-3-0365-5537-9 (Hbk)
ISBN 978-3-0365-5538-6 (PDF)

Cover image courtesy of Canva
(free media image—https://www.canva.com/es_es/politicas-legales/free-media/)

© 2022 by the authors. Articles in this book are Open Access and distributed under the Creative Commons Attribution (CC BY) license, which allows users to download, copy and build upon published articles, as long as the author and publisher are properly credited, which ensures maximum dissemination and a wider impact of our publications.
The book as a whole is distributed by MDPI under the terms and conditions of the Creative Commons license CC BY-NC-ND.

Contents

About the Editors vii

David Facal, Carlos Spuch and Sonia Valladares-Rodriguez
New Trends in Cognitive Aging and Mild Cognitive Impairment
Reprinted from: *Geriatrics* **2022**, *7*, 80, doi:10.3390/geriatrics7040080 1

Silvia Mejia-Arango, Jaqueline Avila, Brian Downer, Marc A. Garcia,
Alejandra Michaels-Obregon, Joseph L. Saenz, Rafael Samper-Ternent and Rebeca Wong
Effect of Demographic and Health Dynamics on Cognitive Status in Mexico between 2001 and 2015: Evidence from the Mexican Health and Aging Study
Reprinted from: *Geriatrics* **2021**, *6*, 63, doi:10.3390/geriatrics6030063 5

Cassandra R. Hatt, Christopher R. Brydges, Jacqueline A. Mogle, Martin J. Sliwinski
and Allison A. M. Bielak
Evaluating the Consistency of Subjective Activity Assessments and Their Relation to Cognition in Older Adults
Reprinted from: *Geriatrics* **2021**, *6*, 74, doi:10.3390/geriatrics6030074 19

Rossella Rizzo, Silvin Paul Knight, James R. C. Davis, Louise Newman, Eoin Duggan,
Rose Anne Kenny and Roman Romero-Ortuno
SART and Individual Trial Mistake Thresholds: Predictive Model for Mobility Decline
Reprinted from: *Geriatrics* **2021**, *6*, 85, doi:10.3390/geriatrics6030085 37

Noreen Orr, Nicola L. Yeo, Sarah G. Dean, Mathew P. White and Ruth Garside
"It Makes You Feel That You Are There": Exploring the Acceptability of Virtual Reality Nature Environments for People with Memory Loss
Reprinted from: *Geriatrics* **2021**, *6*, 27, doi:10.3390/geriatrics6010027 67

Julie D. Ries and Martha Carroll
Feasibility of a Small Group Otago Exercise Program for Older Adults Living with Dementia
Reprinted from: *Geriatrics* **2022**, *7*, 23, doi:10.3390/geriatrics7020023 83

Fulvio Lauretani, Livia Ruffini, Crescenzo Testa, Marco Salvi, Mara Scarlattei,
Giorgio Baldari, Irene Zucchini, Beatrice Lorenzi, Chiara Cattabiani and Marcello Maggio
Cognitive and Behavior Deficits in Parkinson's Disease with Alteration of FDG-PET Irrespective of Age
Reprinted from: *Geriatrics* **2021**, *6*, 110, doi:10.3390/geriatrics6040110 93

José Caamaño-Ponte, Martina Gómez Digón, Mercedes Pereira Pía,
Antonio de la Iglesia Cabezudo, Margarita Echevarría Canoura and David Facal
A Case Study on Polypharmacy and Depression in a 75-Year-Old Woman with Visual Deficits and Charles Bonnet Syndrome
Reprinted from: *Geriatrics* **2021**, *7*, 5, doi:10.3390/geriatrics7010005 101

Carlos Dosil-Díaz, David Facal and Romina Mouriz-Corbelle
Behavioral Interventions in Long-Term Care Facilities during the COVID-19 Pandemic: A Case Study
Reprinted from: *Geriatrics* **2021**, *7*, 1, doi:10.3390/geriatrics7010001 113

About the Editors

David Facal

David Facal received his PhD in Developmental Psychology from the University of Santiago de Compostela (USC) in 2008 with the PhD thesis "Tip Of the Tongue phenomena in aging: Influence of vocabulary, working memory and processing speed", and his master's degree in Clinical Gerontology from the University of A Coruña. He was awarded the Humanitas Award 2007 by the Economical Social Council of the USC for his social work as a psychologist in AGADEA (Alzheimer's Association of Santiago). He has been a Professor at USC's Department of Developmental Psychology since 2010, teaching the bachelor's degree in Pedagogy and the master's degree in Psychogerontology. He has been Coordinator of the USC's master's degree in Psychogerontology since 2020.

Carlos Spuch

Carlos Spuch received his PhD in Neuroscience from the University of Vigo in 2003. He is R4 Researcher of the Translational Neuroscience Group at Galicia Sur Health Research Institute and the GCV17/SAM1 group of CIBERSAM. He has worked in research centres such as the Cajal Institute of the CSIC (Madrid, Spain), the Karolinska Institute (Stockholm, Sweden) and the Hospital 12 de Octubre (Madrid, Spain). Carlos is currently developing different lines of research that are mainly based on the search for biomarkers to diagnose neurodegenerative and neurological diseases such as Alzheimer's disease, depression, schizophrenia, bipolar disorder or multiple sclerosis. He is also working to understand the molecular and neurobiological aspects of schizophrenia and abuse substance disorder, and in different neurorehabilitation therapies (Trisquel or Emotional Training) in patients treated for substance abuse, as well as studying how the therapy works through proteomic studies in saliva. In 2018, Carlos received the Alzheimer Galicia Federation (FAGAL) Award in recognition of his commitment to people with Alzheimer's disease and their families. In 2021, he was appointed as a reference researcher by the Spanish Society of Psychiatry and Mental Health. He is a Lecturer at the University of Vigo and teaches the master's degrees Neuroscience and Nutrition, respectively. He is Coordinator of the Galician Dementia Research Network. Carlos is currently a Member of the Spanish Society of Psychiatry and Mental Health, and since 2022 he has been a Member of the Board of Directors with the National Association of Hospital Research (ANIH).

Sonia Valladares Rodriguez

Sonia Valladares Rodriguez performs her teaching and research work at the USC in the Department of Electronics and Computer Science as an Assistant Professor. Previously, she has worked within the Artificial Intelligence Department of the UNED. Regarding her training, Sonia carried out her doctoral thesis in the field of Biotechnology. The main motivation for her doctoral thesis was the creation of a cognitive assessment mechanism that can be used in the adult population (i.e., over 55 years), as a method of screening and cognitive monitoring for the detection of incipient cognitive problems and to improve the limitations of current tests. Sonia's research was carried out at the University of Vigo where she began her research work in 2008, and involves the use of serious games, machine learning techniques and Information and Communication Technologies. Sonia has published 40 documents included in Scopus, with papers in different Q1 and Q2 journals. Furthermore, she is a Member of the Galician Network for Dementia Research (http://regidem.imaisd.es), and a review board member in different journals and regional research institutions.

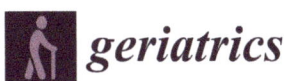

Editorial

New Trends in Cognitive Aging and Mild Cognitive Impairment

David Facal [1], Carlos Spuch [2] and Sonia Valladares-Rodriguez [3,*]

[1] Departamento de Psicoloxía Evolutiva e da Educación, Universidade de Santiago de Compostela, 15782 Santiago de Compostela, Spain; david.facal@usc.es
[2] Translational Neuroscience Group, Galicia Sur Health Research Institute (IIS Galicia Sur), SERGAS-UVIGO, Vigo, and CIBERSAM, ISCIII, 36213 Vigo, Spain; cspuch@uvigo.es
[3] Artificial Intelligence Department, Universidad Nacional de Educación a Distancia (UNED), 28040 Madrid, Spain
* Correspondence: soniavr@dia.uned.es

In this editorial, we aim to highlight some lessons learned in our field and to discuss some open questions regarding the continuum between healthy cognitive aging and dementia. Cognitive aging and cognitive impairment represent two growing realities in the current context of demographic aging, and its study requires new methodological strategies [1]. In this regard, over the last decades, longitudinal studies have gained presence and relevance in the study of cognitive aging. Life-course sociodemographic and health-related conditions can change cognitive profiles of old adults participating in these types of studies across different age cohorts. Mejía-Arango et al. (2021) [2] used data from the 2001 and 2015 years of the Mexican Health and Aging Study (MHAS) to study trends in cognitive impairment and dementia for Mexican older adults aged 60 years or older. They found a higher likelihood of dementia and a lower likelihood of cognitive impairment no dementia (CIND) in 2015 compared to 2001. Controlling for sociodemographic and health factors, these differences remain significant. Differences were found for sex, with living in rural areas and the presence of stroke being associated with increased odds of dementia (versus normal cognitive aging and CIND) in males but not in females, as well as hypertension and diabetes in females but not in males. Being aged 75 years or older was associated with increased odds of CIND (versus normal aging) in males but not in females, and being aged 75 years or older and having healthcare insurance was associated with lower odds of CIND in females but not in males. Regarding the risk of dementia, the authors interpret that those improvements in educational attainment and access to healthcare in Mexican older adults in 2015 compared to 2001 were not enough to compensate for the disadvantages of aging, rural residence, and higher levels of obesity, diabetes, hypertension, or physical disability. Regarding CIND, a higher diagnostic instability was signaled, in accordance with previous research [3,4]. None of the cardiovascular risks or their treatment showed significant effects on CIND odds. In the coming years, the improvement in the detection and prevention of degenerative processes is expected to extend life expectancy with CIND. Professionals in the sector will have to manage populations with a more uncertain cognitive status and with greater needs for stimulation and health promotion.

Another relevant trend in the study of cognitive aging in recent years is the attention paid to subjective cognitive aging. Subjective cognitive decline (SCD) has been proposed as an increased risk cognition characterized by subjective cognitive complaints that cannot be explained by other health conditions, with no evidence of objective cognitive or functional impairment [5]. Pereiro et al. (2021) [5] compared two different thresholds for complaint severity, a stricter criterion considering the 95th percentile and a less strict criterion considering the 5th percentile, showing a higher predictive validity for progression to mild cognitive impairment (MCI) and dementia using the less strict criteria. In this context of increased relevance of subjective information, different authors have started to

Citation: Facal, D.; Spuch, C.; Valladares-Rodriguez, S. New Trends in Cognitive Aging and Mild Cognitive Impairment. *Geriatrics* 2022, 7, 80. https://doi.org/10.3390/geriatrics7040080

Received: 12 July 2022
Accepted: 22 July 2022
Published: 1 August 2022

Publisher's Note: MDPI stays neutral with regard to jurisdictional claims in published maps and institutional affiliations.

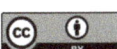

Copyright: © 2022 by the authors. Licensee MDPI, Basel, Switzerland. This article is an open access article distributed under the terms and conditions of the Creative Commons Attribution (CC BY) license (https://creativecommons.org/licenses/by/4.0/).

study the accuracy of subjective reports (i.e., if self-reported or reports provided by proxies present higher predictive validity). Hatt et al. (2021) [6] studied if subjective estimations of activity participation predicted cognitive performance. Subjective estimates of activity are susceptible to different biases, including motivation, attention, emotional experiences, misunderstanding of the activities included in the questionnaires, and misunderstanding of the reported time frames. In total, 199 participants from the Activity Characteristics and Cognition (ACC) study and 170 participants from the TRAnsitions In Later Life (TRAILLs) study were studied. Both samples from different countries reported less activity participation at the weekly level than when they reported activities at a daily basis. Total activity participation did not predict cognitive status, but when activity was grouped by domains, different activity domains (e.g., cognitive, social, and emotional) significantly predicted different cognitive functions.

Cognitive status is closely linked to affective states not only in older adults without pathologies, through their own subjective status, but also in older adults with affective disorders such as depression. Caamaño et al. (2021) [7] highlight the frequent interrelation between organic pathologies, depressive symptomatology, and cognitive function in geriatric patients. The prevalence and intensity of affective disorders have increased due to the COVID-19 pandemic, although not exclusively in the geriatric population. Dosil-Díaz et al. (2021) [8] discuss the management of behavioural and psychological symptoms of dementia (i.e., BPSD) in long-term care centres, considering that the measures taken to control the spread of the virus in these centres dramatically altered the BPSD management interventions and, in general, the social and care activities with the residents. People with BPSD present higher risks of severe infection due to the relationship between frailty and dementia and their difficulties maintaining social isolation or using face masks, among others. In this context, the most relevant strategies were personalized dementia care programs and video call programs allowing social interaction between the resident and their families.

Digital technologies, including computer-based cognitive tests, are more and more common in psychogerontological and psychogeriatric practice. However, this reality is not exempt from complexities associated with its application [9]. For example, in an interesting study about the use of multimodal methods to visualize information obtained from the Sustained Attention to Response Task (SART), Rizzo et al. (2021) [10] proposes a new thresholding method based on the individual trial percentage of mistakes to determine subgroups of old adults with poor SART performance, also considering their age and Timed-Up and Go (TUG) performance. SART is a computerized continuous performance go–no go reaction time task, in which two types of mistakes can be made: commission errors (responding to no go trials) and omission errors (not responding to go trials). This novel multimodal visualization approach can help professional to better identify profiles of high risk of mobility problems in older adults. In this context of the growing use of digital technologies, immersive virtual reality (VR) can be a valuable tool to involve and motivate frail and disabled patients during therapy sessions. Orr et al. (2021) [11] studied the acceptability a series of 5 × 30 second clips of VR nature environments, showing scenes of coast and beaches with natural sounds such as breaking waves, in persons with dementia attending memory cafes. Most of the participants responded positively to the VR scenes, feeling immersed in nature with a sense of "being away" and experiencing new places. In addition, VR is considered to be able to simulate real-life situations to improve ecological validity [12]. Therefore, these technological solutions could act as effective neuropsychological tools for the assessment of everyday cognitive functions, which improve ecological validity and provide a highly enjoyable testing experience. Finally, to conclude, the use of technology in neuropsychological assessment continues to expand and enhance traditional assessment approaches. However, a number of challenges remain, such as, variations in hardware; limited information on psychometric and normative properties for different clinical populations; and the possible influence of computer literacy or other technologies on that population.

As it has been mentioned, mobility has become a central issue not only in general geriatric practice but specifically in the study of cognitive aging. Neurodegenerative diseases such as Parkinson's disease or the functional deterioration caused by pathological aging can cause serious mobility problems in later adulthood. The ability to have proper mobility is closely linked to cognitive functioning itself, with complex networks linking the brain and the locomotor system. Rizzo et al. (2021) [10] showed that participants of the TILDA study with bad SART performances and normal TUG at baseline had higher probability to have a mobility impairment at wave 3 considering both their TUG performance and the risk of becoming a new fall. Difficulties in mobility in pathological aging can be caused neurodegenerative disease itself or vice versa, where a loss of mobility caused by a fall or lack of family care will eventually lead to cognitive impairment that, in many cases, becomes irreversible. This proposal is addressed in the article by Ries and Carroll 2021 [13], which deals with the problem of avoiding the most frequent falls through a prevention program in patients with moderate and severe dementia. They conclude that the type of format of this program determines that participation is optimal, thereby reducing the risk of deterioration caused by a fall or injury.

Complementarily, Lauretani et al. 2021 [14] propose the use of FDG-PET to measure cerebral metabolic rates of glucose in two cases of Parkinson's patients with non-motor symptoms, so that better treatment can be achieved based on metabolic changes and not on age-independent motor deterioration. One of the great challenges facing clinical neuroscience is to detect the presence of cognitive impairment in the early stages before it becomes clinically evident. One of the ways to do this is the research and development of easily accessible molecular biomarkers. In the future, this would allow general screening of at-risk populations and, if positive, further neuroimaging and neuropsychological studies.

The articles included in this Special Issue are just a sample of the current research on cognitive aging and cognitive decline, but they allow us to address this relevant phenomenon considering the close link between cognitive status, health, and functional status in geriatric patients. When we talk about the geriatric population, we are dealing with patients with varied and different neurodegenerative diseases, comorbidities with many pathologies that can cause movement and quality of life deficits (e.g., respiratory, obesity, etc.) and polypharmacy, with a lot of medication that can alter their own quality of life. Regarding mobility, it is a matter of addressing this problem of falls in a preventive way, either through prevention programs, as proposed by Ries and Carroll [13], or by anticipating it through metabolic measures in Parkinson's patients, as proposed by Lauretani et al. [14]. Regarding polypharmacy, it is necessary to understand the complexity of therapeutic approaches and, as highlighted by Caamaño et al. [7], the complexity of the management of these situations in different care systems. In the future, it is expected that the complexity of these situations will increase due to the pressure of population aging, for which the contribution of technologies such as the novel visualization approach proposed by Rizzo et al. (2021) [10] and the natural scenes presented with immersive VR by Orr et al. (2021) [11] will be necessary.

Conflicts of Interest: The authors declare no conflict of interest.

References

1. Facal, D.; Guardía Olmos, J.; Juncos Rabadán, O. Aportaciones metodológicas al estudio de datos de tipo longitudinal en el deterioro cognitivo ligero. *Rev. Esp. Geriatr. Gerontol.* **2014**, *49*, 148–149. [CrossRef] [PubMed]
2. Mejia-Arango, S.; Avila, J.; Downer, B.; Garcia, M.A.; Michaels-Obregon, A.; Saenz, J.L.; Samper-Ternent, R.; Wong, R. Effect of demographic and health dynamics on cognitive status in mexico between 2001 and 2015: Evidence from the mexican health and aging study. *Geriatrics* **2021**, *6*, 63. [CrossRef] [PubMed]
3. Forlenza, O.V.; Diniz, B.S.; Nunes, P.V.; Memória, C.M.; Yassuda, M.S.; Gattaz, W.F. Diagnostic transitions in mild cognitive impairment subtypes. *Int. Psychogeriatr.* **2009**, *21*, 1088–1095. [CrossRef] [PubMed]
4. Facal, D.; Guàrdia-Olmos, J.; Pereiro, A.X.; Lojo-Seoane, C.; Peró, M.; Juncos-Rabadán, O. Using an overlapping time interval strategy to study diagnostic instability in mild cognitive impairment subtypes. *Brain Sci.* **2019**, *9*, 242. [CrossRef] [PubMed]

5. Pereiro, A.X.; Valladares-Rodríguez, S.; Felpete, A.; Lojo-Seoane, C.; Campos-Magdaleno, M.; Mallo, S.C.; Facal, D.; Anido-Rifon, L.; Belleville, S.; Juncos-Rabadán, O. Relevance of complaint severity in predicting the progression of subjective cognitive decline and mild cognitive impairment: A machine learning approach. *J. Alzheimer's Dis.* **2021**, *82*, 1229–1242. [CrossRef] [PubMed]
6. Hatt, C.R.; Brydges, C.R.; Mogle, J.A.; Sliwinski, M.J.; Bielak, A.A. Evaluating the consistency of subjective activity assessments and their relation to cognition in older adults. *Geriatrics* **2021**, *6*, 74. [CrossRef] [PubMed]
7. Caamaño-Ponte, J.; Gómez Digón, M.; Pereira Pía, M.; de la Iglesia Cabezudo, A.; Echevarría Canoura, M.; Facal, D. A case study on polypharmacy and depression in a 75-year-old woman with visual deficits and charles bonnet syndrome. *Geriatrics* **2021**, *7*, 5. [CrossRef] [PubMed]
8. Dosil-Díaz, C.; Facal, D.; Mouriz-Corbelle, R. Behavioral interventions in long-term care facilities during the COVID-19 pandemic: A case study. *Geriatrics* **2021**, *7*, 1. [CrossRef] [PubMed]
9. Parsey, C.M.; Schmitter-Edgecombe, M. Applications of technology in neuropsychological assessment. *Clin. Neuropsychol.* **2013**, *27*, 1328–1361. [CrossRef] [PubMed]
10. Rizzo, R.; Knight, S.P.; Davis, J.R.; Newman, L.; Duggan, E.; Kenny, R.A.; Romero-Ortuno, R. SART and Individual Trial Mistake Thresholds: Predictive Model for Mobility Decline. *Geriatrics* **2021**, *6*, 85. [CrossRef] [PubMed]
11. Orr, N.; Yeo, N.L.; Dean, S.G.; White, M.P.; Garside, R. "It makes you feel that you are there": Exploring the acceptability of virtual reality nature environments for people with memory loss. *Geriatrics* **2021**, *6*, 27. [CrossRef] [PubMed]
12. Kourtesis, P.; Collina, S.; Doumas, L.A.; MacPherson, S.E. Validation of the Virtual Reality Everyday Assessment Lab (VR-EAL): An immersive virtual reality neuropsychological battery with enhanced ecological validity. *J. Int. Neuropsychol. Soc.* **2021**, *27*, 181–196. [CrossRef] [PubMed]
13. Ries, J.D.; Carroll, M. Feasibility of a Small Group Otago Exercise Program for Older Adults Living with Dementia. *Geriatrics* **2022**, *7*, 23. [CrossRef] [PubMed]
14. Lauretani, F.; Longobucco, Y.; Ravazzoni, G.; Gallini, E.; Salvi, M.; Maggio, M. Imaging the Functional Neuroanatomy of Parkinson's Disease: Clinical Applications and Future Directions. *Int. J. Environ. Res. Public Health* **2021**, *18*, 2356. [CrossRef] [PubMed]

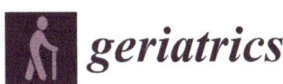

Article

Effect of Demographic and Health Dynamics on Cognitive Status in Mexico between 2001 and 2015: Evidence from the Mexican Health and Aging Study

Silvia Mejia-Arango [1], Jaqueline Avila [2], Brian Downer [3], Marc A. Garcia [4], Alejandra Michaels-Obregon [3], Joseph L. Saenz [5], Rafael Samper-Ternent [3] and Rebeca Wong [3,*]

1. Department of Population Studies, El Colegio de la Frontera Norte, Tijuana 22560, Baja California, Mexico; smejia@colef.mx
2. Center for Alcohol and Addiction Studies, School of Public Health, Brown University, Providence, RI 02912, USA; jaqueline_avila@brown.edu
3. Sealy Center on Aging, University of Texas Medical Branch, Galveston, TX 77555, USA; brdowner@utmb.edu (B.D.); almichae@utmb.edu (A.M.-O.); rasamper@utmb.edu (R.S.-T.)
4. Department of Sociology, Institute for Ethnic Studies, University of Nebraska, Lincoln, NE 68588-0324, USA; marcagarcia@unl.edu
5. Leonard Davis School of Gerontology, University of Southern California, Los Angeles, CA 90089, USA; saenzj@usc.edu
* Correspondence: rewong@utmb.edu; Tel.: +1-(409)-266-9661

Abstract: Sources of health disparities such as educational attainment, cardiovascular risk factors, and access to health care affect cognitive impairment among older adults. To examine the extent to which these counteracting changes affect cognitive aging over time among Mexican older adults, we examine how sociodemographic factors, cardiovascular diseases, and their treatment relate to changes in cognitive function of Mexican adults aged 60 and older between 2001 and 2015. Self and proxy respondents were classified as dementia, cognitive impairment no dementia (CIND), and normal cognition. We use logistic regression models to examine the trends in dementia and CIND for men and women aged 60 years or older using pooled national samples of 6822 individuals in 2001 and 10,219 in 2015, and sociodemographic and health variables as covariates. We found higher likelihood of dementia and a lower risk of CIND in 2015 compared to 2001. These results remain after adjusting for sociodemographic factors, cardiovascular diseases, and their treatment. The improvements in educational attainment, treatment of diabetes and hypertension, and better access to health care in 2015 compared to 2001 may not have been enough to counteract the combined effects of aging, rural residence disadvantage, and higher risks of cardiovascular disease among older Mexican adults.

Keywords: cognitive aging; epidemiology; healthcare disparities; minority health

1. Introduction

Over the past 15 years, research on cognitive impairment and dementia in low- and middle-income countries has increased as the potential for a significant increase in dementia burden in faster-aging populations occurs [1]. Data from the Mexican Health and Aging Study (MHAS), a nationally representative panel study, has been widely used by researchers interested in cognitive aging. Several studies [2,3] have found that older age, fewer years of education, female sex, and rural residence are strong sociodemographic predictors of cognitive impairment. Highly prevalent chronic diseases among Mexican adults, such as hypertension, stroke, and diabetes, are associated with cognitive impairment [4,5].

In Mexico, it is well established that more recent cohorts of older adults aged 60 and older have higher educational achievement [6]. However, as a group, the more recent cohorts also have a higher prevalence of obesity, diabetes, hypertension, and physical disability [7,8]. This combination of change in key socioeconomic factors and health risks of the older adult population is quite evident by comparing cohorts who are only ten years apart, for example, those 60 and older in 2001 and 2012 [9–11]. Over the same decade, the country implemented reforms in social protection programs that benefit older adults, most notably the gradual implementation of Seguro Popular, a public health insurance program seeking to achieve universal health care, which started circa 2003 [12]. Previous work reports noticeable gains in the share of older adults with health insurance [13], the use of preventive care tests [4], and improved awareness and treatment of chronic conditions such as hypertension and diabetes [10]. Gender-specific associations have shown that the availability of health insurance is more likely to increase medical service utilization in women than in men [14].

This combination of relatively fast changes in sociodemographic and population health profiles of older adults likely contributed to changes in the burden of cognitive impairment and dementia. In high-income countries, despite increasing trends in cardiovascular health, previous studies report a decline in dementia incidence or prevalence among older adults, which they attribute largely to improvements in treatments of cardiovascular risk factors and rising levels of education [15–17]. In Mexico, it is unclear how the important sociodemographic and health-related changes previously mentioned, which occurred mostly in the last two decades [18], are associated with changes in cognitive aging among older adults. We seek to fill this gap by comparing data from MHAS collected at two different points in time: 2001 and 2015.

The aim of this manuscript was to examine how sociodemographic factors, cardiovascular diseases, and their treatment relate to the cognitive status of Mexican adults aged 60 and older between 2001 and 2015. We hypothesized that higher educational achievement and more access to health care, including treatment of cardiovascular diseases, would imply a trend towards better cognitive function. On the other hand, survival to older ages and a higher prevalence of chronic diseases among survivors would indicate a trend towards worse cognitive function. These counter-acting influences mean that the overall time trend in cognitive function is ambiguous. Our approach sought to inform the extent to which the future burden of cognitive aging in Mexico can be potentially addressed with health interventions targeting better prevention, management, and treatment of highly prevalent chronic conditions.

2. Materials and Methods

2.1. Participants

The MHAS is a longitudinal cohort study of adults aged 50 and older in Mexico with national and urban-rural representation. The first wave was in 2001 with a sample of adults born in 1951 or earlier. Four follow-up waves were in 2003, 2012, 2015, and 2018 [19]. The study follows participants until their death. Additional refresher cohorts include those born in 1952–1961, added in 2012, and those born in 1962–1968, added in 2018. We used data from the 2001 and 2015 years for the current study [20]. The MHAS study seeks to complete interviews directly with the participants, but interviews by proxy are possible in cases of extreme disability, illness, or temporary absence. Figure 1 illustrates the sample selection process in both waves for the current analyses. We included all participants aged 60 and over who answered the survey through a direct or proxy interview. We selected individuals who completed at least two of five cognitive tasks included in the MHAS cognitive battery from those with a direct interview. Participants who refused the full cognitive assessment and those who completed only one task were excluded from our analysis (n = 334 in 2001 and n = 86 in 2015). The excluded participants tend to be male, older, and less educated. From proxy participants, we excluded those with incomplete information (n = 2 in 2001 and n = 2 in 2015). The final sample was 6822 participants in 2001 and 10,219 in 2015, which we treat as two cross-sections for our comparison. Individuals present in both cohorts were 2951, while 3871 were included only in 2001 and 8268 only in 2015.

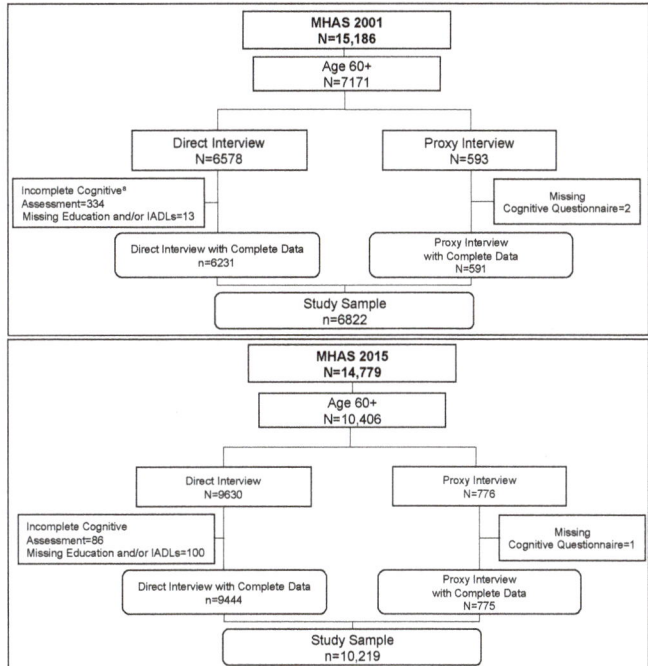

Figure 1. Flowchart of the Sample Selection for the 2001 and 2015 Cohorts. Note: Flowchart of sample selection in 2001 ($n = 6822$) and 2015 ($n = 10,219$). [a] More cognitive assessments were incomplete in 2001 compared to 2015 because more of the 2001 participants refused to participate in the cognitive assessment because they spoke only the Indigenous language. In 2015, these cases were no longer pursued.

2.2. Definition of Cognitive Categories

A team of cognitive researchers collaborated with MHAS investigators to adopt a conceptual model for cognitive aging. We identified factors that influenced cognition and standardized the process to classify individuals into three cognitive categories: normal cognition, cognitive impairment no dementia (CIND), and dementia, using a comprehensive set of variables from the MHAS study. We summarize our framework in Figure 2 and highlight the established relationships between different factors that affect cognitive status. Figure 2 starts with three contextual levels in which cognitive aging occurs, namely: (1) The macro-social context, which includes the demographic and epidemiologic transitions; (2) The institutional and public policy context, which refers to the government and institutional support systems; and (3) The environmental context, which refers to group characteristics such as residence, population size, migration, and environmental exposures. These contextual aspects provide relevant information to understand potential differences between populations [21].

Underlying the process of cognitive aging are life-course socioeconomic and health conditions, current health conditions (cerebrovascular conditions, health behaviors, and health care), and genetic factors associated with normal or pathological (neurodegenerative disease) brain changes during aging [22]. Brain and cognitive reserve are key concepts to capture potential differences in the brain's structural aspects and compensatory mechanisms that shape how the brain copes with age-related changes and pathology such as dementia [23]. These concepts include characteristics such as anatomical features of the brain structure, and the brain function indicators such as educational and occupational attainment.

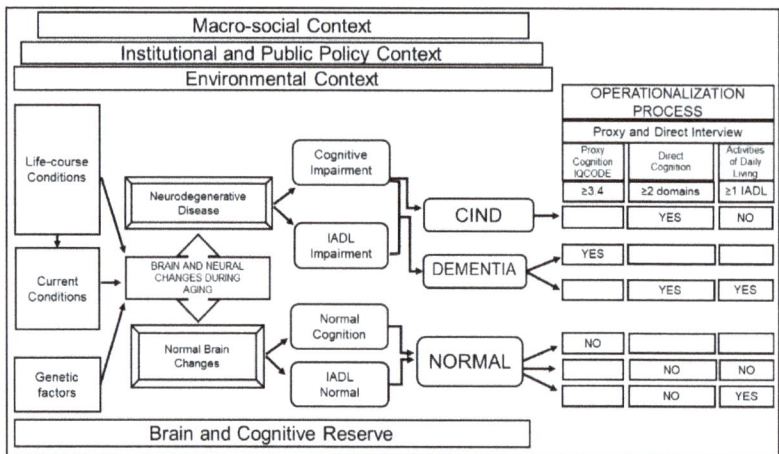

Figure 2. Conceptual framework for the definition of cognitive status in MHAS. Note: Framework showing how normal or pathological brain changes during aging are influenced by different factors (e.g., contextual, life-course, current conditions, genetic, brain reserve) and result in cognitive and functional symptoms (normal or impaired) which define cognitive status classification (CIND, dementia or normal cognition). Following this framework, data from MHAS is used to operationalize each category. Abbreviations: MHAS, Mexican Health and Aging Study; CIND, cognitive impairment no dementia; IADL, instrumental activities of daily living; IQCODE, Informant Questionnaire on Cognitive Decline in the Elderly.

Following the criteria for preclinical and clinical phases of all-cause dementia recommended by the National Institute on Aging and the Alzheimer's Association [24,25] and prior literature from population studies [26], we classified individuals into three groups based on their cognitive status and the ability to function independently in instrumental activities of daily living (IADLs). Individuals with a neurodegenerative disease may exhibit cognitive impairment and limitations in IADLs (dementia) or cognitive impairment, but no limitations in IADLs (CIND). On the other hand, individuals with normal brain changes will have normal cognition and no limitations in IADLs, or normal cognition and impairment in IADLs due to physical limitations.

The operationalization process linking these categories to the MHAS study variables was as follows: (1) Dementia: self-respondents with impairment in two or more cognitive domains and one or more IADL limitations, or proxy respondents with scores above the cut-point (≥ 3.4) on the Informant Questionnaire on Cognitive Decline in the Elderly (IQCODE) [27]; (2) CIND: self-respondents with impairment in two or more cognitive domains and no IADL functional limitations; (3) Normal cognition: self-respondents with normal cognitive function and no IADL limitations or impairment in IADLs due to physical limitations, and proxy respondents with IQCODE score below the cut-point (< 3.4).

2.3. Cognitive Measures

The MHAS assessment in self-respondents uses a cognitive assessment adapted from the Cross-Cultural Cognitive Evaluation (CCCE) [28] in five cognitive domains: verbal learning (eight-word list presented during three trials), verbal memory (delayed recall of eight-word list), attention (visual scan of target stimuli), constructional praxis (copy of a figure), and visual memory (delayed recall of figure). Cognitive impairment in each domain was defined as a score 1.5 standard deviations (SD) below the mean based on reference norms by age and years of education [29]. The MHAS uses the adapted CCCE mainly because of its cross-cultural attributes, including ease of application among low-education groups.

For respondents represented by a proxy, cognitive function was assessed through the brief version of the IQCODE [27], a 16-item questionnaire on cognitive decline in the elderly, rated on a 5-point scale from 1 "much improved" to 5 "much worse." An informant who knew about the participant's daily functioning, usually a spouse or adult child or caregiver, rated the participant's cognitive status compared to how it was two years earlier. We used a cut-point of 3.4 and above to classify dementia, as the scale has a reported sensitivity of 85% and a specificity of 80% in population-based cohorts [30].

2.4. Covariates

Following previous research [3,8,18,26,31,32], we included the following covariates shown to have an association with cognitive impairment. Sociodemographic variables: sex (male/female); age used as a continuous or categorical variable (60 to 74 years and ≥75 years); years of formal education as a continuous or categorical variable (0 years, 1 to 6 years, and ≥7 years) following the formative periods in the Mexican education system; and area of residence as a categorical variable (rural for ≤2500 people and urban >2500 people). Cardiovascular risk factors: Self-reported stroke, diabetes, heart disease, and hypertension (all yes/no). Cardiovascular treatment: Among those who have each condition, self-reported use of medications for stroke, diabetes (either oral medications or insulin), heart disease, and hypertension (all yes/no). Body mass index (BMI); calculated with self-reported weight [kilograms] divided by height [meters and centimeters] squared [kilogram per square meter] categorized as underweight (<18.5), normal (18.5–24.9), overweight (25.0–29.9), obese (≥30) based on the World Health Organization (WHO) classification. Health insurance: Self-reported dichotomous variable (yes-no).

2.5. Statistical Analysis

For descriptive analyses, we examined differences in covariates between total participants in the 2001 and 2015 cohorts and stratified by cognitive status using a t-test or χ^2 test as appropriate. Because education is a critical covariate of cognitive aging, and there are important gender differences in educational achievement in Mexico, we present the multivariate results for the total analytical sample and results stratified by sex. For multivariable analyses, we pooled data from both years (2001 and 2015) and estimated two logistic regression models. The first model included the dichotomous dependent variable indicating if an individual had dementia versus no dementia (normal cognition and CIND); in the second model, CIND versus normal cognition was the dependent variable. In each model, we included a linear trend variable with the value 0 in 2001 and 1 in 2015. An odds ratio less or greater than 1 in the trend variable would indicate a decrease or an increase, respectively, in the likelihood of dementia and CIND in 2015 compared to 2001. We estimated an unadjusted model with the trend variable only and a fully adjusted model including all covariates: sociodemographic factors, BMI, each of four cardiovascular diseases, treatment for each disease, and health insurance. We tested for interactions between each independent variable and the trend variable to assess if the effect of each covariate was different in 2015 compared to 2001. We used IBM SPSS Statistics, Version 25.0 (IBM Corp., Armonk, NY, USA) for statistical analyses.

3. Results

3.1. Trends in Cognitive Status

Roughly 70–80% of the sample was classified as normal cognition (70.6% in 2001 and 79.1% in 2015). CIND individuals represented 23.3% (95% Confidence Interval [CI], 22.2–24.4) of the sample in 2001 and 13.5% (95% CI, 12.8–14.3) in 2015 ($p < 0.001$). Those classified with dementia were 6.1% (95% CI, 5.5–6.7) in 2001 and 7.3% (95% CI, 6.8–7.9) in the 2015 sample ($p = 0.002$). Table S1 in the Supplementary Material shows the distribution of covariates by cognition status for both years.

3.2. Trends in Sociodemographic Characteristics

Table 1 shows descriptive characteristics of Mexican adults aged 60 and older in the years 2001 and 2015. Results were weighted to represent the national populations of older adults in the corresponding year. Compared with 2001, the cohort for 2015 contained a significantly larger proportion of individuals aged 75 years and older and this cohort had a higher average age. The share of women increased from 52.4% in 2001 to 54.8% in 2015 ($p = 0.002$). On average, older adults in 2015 had one more year of education compared to those in 2001 ($p < 0.001$). The proportion of individuals with no schooling decreased from 36.0% in 2001 to 24.0% in 2015 ($p < 0.001$), and the share of participants with seven or more years of education increased from 13.7% in 2001 to 22.9% in 2015 ($p < 0.001$). The absolute increase in educational achievement years was larger for men than for women and larger for those aged 60–74 compared to those aged 75 and older (data not shown). The proportion of individuals living in rural or urban areas did not differ significantly between 2001 and 2015.

Table 1. Characteristics of participants aged 60 and older of the 2001 and 2015 cohorts [a].

	2001	2015	
	n = 6822	n = 10219	p Value
Age, y			
60–74 years	5224 (74.5)	7073 (72.5)	<0.001
≥75 years	1598 (25.5)	3146 (27.5)	<0.001
Mean (SD)	69.3 (7.5)	71.2 (7.9)	<0.001
Sex			
Male	3169 (47.6)	4496 (45.2)	0.002
Female	3653 (52.4)	5723 (54.8)	
Education, y			
No schooling	2138 (36.0)	2142 (24.0)	<0.001
1–6 years	3646 (50.3)	5541 (52.9)	0.31
≥7 years	1038 (13.7)	2536 (22.9)	<0.001
Mean (SD)	3.6 (3.9)	4.9 (4.5)	<0.001
Residence			
Urban	4936 (57.8)	7267 (60.5)	0.08
Rural	1886 (42.2)	2952 (39.5)	
Cardiovascular conditions			
Hypertension	2876 (41.3)	5354 (50.3)	<0.001
Diabetes	1188 (16.8)	2686 (24.9)	<0.001
Heart attack	298 (3.3)	477 (3.8)	0.37
Stroke	254 (3.5)	293 (2.6)	0.002
CVD Treatment [b]			
Hypertension	2190 (76.3)	4738 (85.9)	<0.001
Diabetes	1030 (87.6)	2499 (93.2)	<0.001
Heart attack	211 (66.8)	341 (70.7)	0.95
Stroke	141 (53.4)	153 (46.9)	0.44
BMI			
18.5–24.9 (Normal)	2491 (38.7)	3511 (34.8)	0.004
<18.5 (Underweight)	158 (3.5)	185 (2.2)	0.03
25.0–29.9 (Overweight)	2983 (41.5)	4331 (42.9)	0.08
≥30 (Obese)	1183 (16.3)	2182 (20.1)	<0.001
Health insurance (yes)	4287 (56.9)	9376 (90.4)	<0.001

Notes: Characteristics are presented as n (%) unless otherwise indicated. Values in parenthesis are weighted % derived using sampling weights of the MHAS. [a] The reported p value is for χ^2 or t test for a significant difference in proportion or mean between years. [b] Cardiovascular treatment for those with each condition. Abbreviations: BMI, body mass index; CVD, cardiovascular conditions; SD, standard deviation.

3.3. Trends in Cardiovascular Risks and Treatment

The prevalence of some, but not all, cardiovascular conditions among Mexican adults aged 60 or older was higher in 2015 compared to 2001. Diabetes increased from 16.8% to 24.9% ($p < 0.001$). Similarly, hypertension increased from 41.3% in 2001 to 50.3% in 2015

($p < 0.001$). Conversely, the prevalence of stroke decreased from 3.5% in 2001 to 2.6% in 2015 ($p = 0.002$), whereas heart disease prevalence did not change significantly. Regarding treatment among older adults, the proportion of participants with hypertension treatment increased from 76.3% in 2001 to 85.9% in 2015 ($p < 0.001$). Similarly, diabetes treatment increased from 87.6% to 93.2% ($p < 0.001$). Heart attack and stroke treatment were similar in the two periods.

Based on BMI classification, the share of individuals in the normal range decreased from 38.7% in 2001 to 34.8% ($p = 0.004$) in 2015. The underweight percentage also decreased slightly, from 3.5% to 2.2% ($p = 0.03$). The fraction of overweight remained the same between the two periods, while obesity increased from 16.3% in 2001 to 20.1% in 2015 ($p < 0.001$). Compared with 2001, the proportion of individuals with health insurance increased significantly, from 56.9% to 90.4% in 2015 ($p < 0.001$).

3.4. Regression Results

Table 2 shows the results of a fully adjusted logistic regression model, for the overall sample and stratified by sex, with dementia (versus normal cognition or CIND) as the outcome variable, and using pooled 2001 and 2015 data. The trend variable in the first row of the table represents the adjusted odds ratio (OR) of dementia in 2015 compared with 2001. The unadjusted OR of the trend variable (results not shown) showed a significantly higher likelihood of dementia in 2015 compared to 2001 for the overall sample (OR [95% confidence interval]: (1.23 [1.08–1.39], $p = 0.001$) and for men (1.37 [1.12–1.69], $p = 0.002$), but not significantly so for women (1.13 [0.97–1.32], $p = 0.118$)). After controlling for the effect of sociodemographic factors, cardiovascular conditions, treatment of cardiovascular conditions, BMI, and health insurance, both the overall sample and males continued to show higher odds of dementia in 2015. For females, the odds of dementia were also higher, now reaching statistical significance.

Table 2. Odds ratios for dementia, overall and stratified by sex [a].

	Overall		Males		Females	
	OR (95% CI)	p Value	OR (95% CI)	p Value	OR (95% CI)	p Value
Trend (2015 vs. 2001)	1.27 (1.10–1.47)	0.001	1.33 (1.09–1.69)	0.020	1.24 (1.03–1.49)	0.020
Sex, Female	1.50 (1.32–1.72)	<0.001	NA		NA	
Age, y						
60–74 years	1 [Reference]		1 [Reference]		1 [Reference]	
≥75 years	4.53 (3.97–5.17)	<0.001	4.72 (3.78–5.90)	<0.001	4.34 (3.68–5.13)	<0.001
Education, y						
0 years	1.93 (1.56–2.40)	<0.001	2.13 (1.49–3.05)	<0.001	1.81 (1.38–2.37)	<0.001
1–6 years	1.36 (1.11–1.66)	0.003	1.40 (1.00–1.95)	0.05	1.32 (1.02–1.70)	0.03
≥7 years	1 [Reference]		1 [Reference]		1 [Reference]	
Residence						
Urban	1 [Reference]		1 [Reference]		1 [Reference]	
Rural	1.04 (0.90–1.20)	0.57	1.36 (1.09–1.71)	0.006	0.87 (0.72–1.05)	0.16
Cardiovascular disease						
Hypertension	1.27 (1.00–1.61)	0.05	0.74 (0.46–1.20)	0.23	1.55 (1.17–2.05)	0.002
Diabetes	1.60 (1.08–2.36)	0.02	1.56 (0.82–2.98)	0.17	1.68 (1.02–2.77)	0.04
Heart disease	1.46 (0.94–2.27)	0.09	1.46 (0.76–2.81)	0.25	1.46 (0.79–2.68)	0.22
Stroke	2.18 (1.52–3.13)	<0.001	3.80 (2.21–6.54)	<0.001	1.55 (0.95–2.51)	0.08
BMI						
Underweight (<18.5)	1.46 (1.06–2.01)	0.02	1.68 (1.01–2.79)	0.04	1.36 (0.90–2.07)	0.14
Normal (18.5–24.9)	1 [Reference]		1 [Reference]		1 [Reference]	
Overweight (25.0–29.9)	0.72 (0.63–0.83)	<0.001	0.70 (0.55–0.88)	0.002	0.73 (0.61–0.88)	0.001
Obese (≥30.0)	0.63 (0.52–0.77)	<0.001	0.55 (0.38–0.82)	0.003	0.66 (0.52–0.83)	0.001

Table 2. Cont.

	Overall		Males		Females	
	OR (95% CI)	p Value	OR (95% CI)	p Value	OR (95% CI)	p Value
CVD Treatment [b]						
Hypertension	0.83 (0.65–1.06)	0.15	1.33 (0.81–2.19)	0.25	0.71 (0.54–0.94)	0.02
Diabetes	0.91 (0.60–1.36)	0.65	1.10 (0.56–2.14)	0.77	0.80 (0.48–1.34)	0.41
Heart disease	0.99 (0.59–1.68)	0.98	1.08 (0.51–2.32)	0.82	0.93 (0.45–1.92)	0.86
Stroke	3.24 (2.08–5.05)	<0.001	2.13 (1.11–4.09)	0.022	4.04 (2.18–7.46)	<0.001
Health care insurance [c]	0.75 (0.63–0.89)	0.001	0.94 (0.71–1.26)	0.72	0.66 (0.54–0.82)	<0.001

Note. [a] Adjusted odds ratios were derived using logistic regression models with pooled data from 2001 (n = 6791) and 2015 (n = 10,215) for the overall sample; 2001 (n = 3155) and 2015 (n = 4494) for males; 2001 (n = 3636) and 2015 (n = 5271) for females. The dependent variable was dementia compared to normal cognition or CIND. [b] Cardiovascular treatment for those with each condition. [c] Health care insurance for those with insurance. Abbreviations: OR = odds ratio; CI = confidence interval; BMI = Body Mass Index; CVD, cardiovascular disease; NA, not applicable.

For the overall sample, being female (1.50 [1.32–1.72], $p < 0.001$), being 75 years or older (4.53 [3.97–5.17], $p < 0.001$), and low educational achievement were associated with a significantly higher odds of dementia. Compared to having seven or more years of education, individuals with no schooling (1.93 [1.56–2.40], $p < 0.001$) and those with one to six years of education (1.36 [1.11–1.66], $p = 0.003$) had a higher likelihood of dementia. Higher odds of dementia also were associated with a history of hypertension, diabetes, and stroke. Being overweight (0.72 [0.63–0.83], $p < 0.001$) or obese (0.63 [0.52–0.77], $p < 0.001$) was associated with lower odds of dementia compared to having normal BMI.

The results showed noticeable differences when stratified by sex. Older age and lower education were associated with higher odds of dementia for both males and females. Living in rural areas was associated with increased odds of dementia in males (1.36 [1.09–1.71], $p = 0.006$) but not in females. Odds were significantly increased for those with hypertension (1.55 [1.17–2.05], $p = 0.002$) and diabetes (1.68 [1.02–2.77], $p = 0.04$) in females but not in males, while stroke was significant only in males (3.80 [2.21–6.4], $p < 0.001$). Similar to the overall sample results, being overweight or obese was associated with lower odds of dementia in males and females compared to those with normal BMI.

Regarding self-reported treatment, the effect of diabetes and heart attack treatment was not significant, although both were associated with lower odds of dementia; for hypertension treatment, the association was significant only in females (0.71 [0.54–0.94], $p = 0.02$) but not in males. Receiving treatment for stroke was associated with a significantly *higher* odds of dementia, in both males (2.13 [1.11–4.09], $p = 0.02$) and females (4.04 [2.18–7.46], $p < 0.001$). Having health care insurance was associated with lower odds of dementia in females (0.66 [0.54–0.82], $p < 0.001$) but not in males.

We tested for an interaction effect between each covariate and the trend variable (results not shown), controlling for the main effects of all the other covariates. Hypertension treatment was associated with significantly lower odds of dementia in 2015 (0.51 [0.29–0.90], $p = 0.02$) compared with 2001 in females, but not in males. No other interactions with the trend variable were significant.

Table 3 shows the results of a logistic regression model for the overall sample and stratified by sex with CIND (versus normal cognition) as the outcome variable, using pooled 2001 and 2015 data. The unadjusted OR of the trend variable (results not shown) showed a significant decline in the likelihood of CIND between 2001 and 2015 for the overall sample (OR [95% CI]: (0.52 [0.48–0.56], $p < 0.001$), for men (0.62 [0.55–0.69], $p < 0.001$), and for women (0.43 [0.38–0.49], $p < 0.001$)). After controlling for all covariates, these effects of the trend variable remained the same.

Table 3. Odds ratios for CIND, overall and stratified by sex [a].

	Overall		Males		Females	
	OR (95% CI)	p Value	OR (95% CI)	p Value	OR (95% CI)	p Value
Trend (2015 vs. 2001)	0.53 (0.49–0.58)	<0.001	0.61 (0.54–0.69)	<0.001	0.46 (0.41–0.53)	<0.001
Sex, Male	1.33 (1.22–1.44)	<0.001	NA		NA	
Age, y						
60–74 years	1 [Reference]		1 [Reference]		1 [Reference]	
≥75 years	1.01 (0.92–1.12)	0.70	1.26 (1.11–1.44)	<0.001	0.78 (0.68–0.91)	0.001
Education, y						
0 years	0.83 (0.72–0.94)	0.006	0.76 (0.63–0.91)	0.004	0.89 (0.74–1.07)	0.23
1–6 years	0.95 (0.85–1.06)	0.38	1.00 (0.86–1.16)	0.97	0.90 (0.77–1.06)	0.22
≥7 years	1 [Reference]		1 [Reference]		1 [Reference]	
Residence						
Urban	1 [Reference]		1 [Reference]		1 [Reference]	
Rural	1.36 (1.23–1.49)	<0.001	1.36 (1.19–1.54)	<0.001	1.36 (1.18–1.56)	<0.001
Cardiovascular disease						
Hypertension	0.98 (0.83–1.14)	0.80	0.95 (0.76–1.19)	0.68	0.98 (0.78–1.22)	0.86
Diabetes	1.10 (0.83–1.46)	0.50	1.20 (0.82–1.75)	0.33	0.98 (0.63–1.52)	0.93
Heart disease	0.69 (0.46–1.05)	0.09	0.78 (0.47–1.29)	0.34	0.53 (0.25–1.11)	0.09
Stroke	0.71 (0.48–1.06)	0.09	0.61 (0.32–1.14)	0.12	0.80 (0.48–1.33)	0.40
BMI						
Underweight (<18.5)	1.05 (0.79–1.40)	0.72	1.19 (0.79–1.78)	0.39	0.94 (0.62–1.42)	0.77
Normal (18.5–24.9)	1 [Reference]		1 [Reference]		1 [Reference]	
Overweight (25.0–29.9)	0.88 (0.80–0.96)	0.008	0.89 (0.78–1.01)	0.07	0.86 (0.75–0.98)	0.03
Obese (≥30.0)	0.70 (0.62–0.79)	<0.001	0.75 (0.62–0.90)	0.002	0.67 (0.56–0.79)	<0.001
CVD Treatment [b]						
Hypertension	0.97 (0.83–1.14)	0.77	1.02 (0.80–1.29)	0.84	0.95 (0.76–1.19)	0.70
Diabetes	0.98 (0.73–1.32)	0.91	0.92 (0.62–1.37)	0.70	1.07 (0.68–1.70)	0.74
Heart disease	1.18 (0.73–1.92)	0.48	1.06 (0.58–1.92)	0.84	1.49 (0.64–3.45)	0.35
Stroke	1.56 (0.92–2.64)	0.09	1.93 (0.90–4.11)	0.08	1.30 (0.60–2.83)	0.50
Health care insurance [c]	0.85 (0.77–0.95)	0.004	0.87 (0.75–1.01)	0.07	0.82 (0.70–0.95)	0.01

Notes: [a] Adjusted odds ratios were derived using logistic regression models with pooled data from 2001 ($n = 6382$) and 2015 ($n = 9464$) for the overall sample; 2001 ($n = 3012$) and 2015 ($n = 4214$) for males; 2001 ($n = 3370$) and 2015 ($n = 5250$) for females. The dependent variable was CIND compared to normal cognition. [b] Cardiovascular treatment for those with each condition. [c] Health care insurance for those with insurance. Abbreviations: CIND = cognitive impairment no dementia; OR = odds ratio; CI = confidence interval; BMI = Body Mass Index. CVD, cardiovascular disease; NA, not applicable.

For the overall sample, the fully adjusted model showed that being male (1.33 [1.22–1.44], $p < 0.001$) and living in rural areas (1.36 [1.23–1.49], $p < 0.001$) were associated with higher odds of CIND. Having no formal schooling (0.83 [0.72–0.94], $p = 0.006$), being overweight (0.88 [0.80–0.96], $p = 0.008$) or obese (0.70 [0.62–0.79], $p < 0.001$), and having access to health care (0.85 [0.77–0.95], $p = 0.004$) were all associated with lower odds of CIND. The results stratified by sex showed noticeable differences. For males, the odds of CIND were higher in those aged 75 years and older (1.26 [1.11–1.44], $p < 0.001$), while for females, the odds of CIND were lower in the same age group (0.78 [0.68–0.91], $p < 0.001$). Having no formal schooling was significantly associated with lower odds of CIND in males (0.76 [0.63–0.91], $p = 0.004$) but not in females. Having health care insurance was associated with lower odds of CIND in females (0.82 [0.70–0.95], $p = 0.01$) but not in males. Other results were similar for men and women; the odds of CIND were significantly higher for rural residence in males (1.36 [1.19–1.54], $p < 0.001$) and females (1.36 [1.18–1.56], $p < 0.001$). Compared to those with normal weight, the odds of CIND were lower for obesity in males (0.75 [0.62–0.90], $p = 0.002$) and females (0.67 [0.56–0.79], $p < 0.001$). Of note, there were no significant effects ($p > 0.05$) on the odds of CIND associated with any of the cardiovascular health conditions or the treatment of these conditions for the overall sample or for the sample stratified by sex.

We tested for an interaction effect between each covariate and the trend variable, controlling for the main effects of all the other covariates. We found significant interactions with the sociodemographic variables (sex, age, education, rural residence), implying that the effect of these variables on CIND was higher in 2015 compared to their effect in 2001. No other interactions were significant.

4. Discussion

Our data confirmed three important changes that occurred during the 14-year period that may have affected the burden of cognitive aging. The composition of older Mexican adults changed towards their being older and more educated, although a gender gap in education favoring men was still evident. Other major changes were a much higher level of health insurance coverage and a higher prevalence of chronic health conditions, all consistent with previous research [18,32,33]. Because of these changes, it is possible that participants in 2015 were more aware of cardiovascular conditions than participants in 2001.

With this context of sociodemographic, health conditions, and health care changes, we used the cognitive status classification to examine whether the likelihood of cognitive impairment was different in 2015 compared to 2001 among adults aged 60 and older stratified by sex, and the effect of these covariates. Our multivariate models showed a robust result of higher odds of dementia and lower odds of CIND for both men and women in 2015 compared to 2001. Factors associated with a higher likelihood of dementia, such as older age, some cardiovascular risks, and rural residence, were operating in both years. Other factors associated with lower odds of dementia counteracted, such as higher educational achievement, being overweight and obese, and having health insurance. After all these factors were taken into account, a higher likelihood of dementia remained in 2015 for both men and women. Further, our results showed that the effect of these factors on the likelihood of dementia was overall similar for both years.

Our results for dementia stratified by sex also convey noteworthy differences regarding the covariates. The detrimental effects of rural residence and stroke history were significant only for men, while the effects of hypertension and diabetes were evident only for women. The beneficial influence of health insurance was significant for women but not for men, a finding which was consistent with previous literature [14]. This finding is also consistent with our result that hypertension treatment was higher only for women, and the effect appeared to be higher in 2015 compared to 2001. This set of results points to future research regarding gender disparities in the disease risks associated with dementia in Mexican men and women.

Surprisingly, stroke treatment showed a significant association with higher odds of dementia in both males and females. Further analyses showed that the time following stroke was shorter (five years or less) among those with cognitive impairment who were using medication compared to those with no treatment, suggesting a higher rate of post-stroke complications [34].

The covariates for the likelihood of CIND were quite different from those for dementia: only sociodemographic factors such as rural residence and obesity were associated with higher likelihood of CIND, and none of the cardiovascular risks or their treatment showed significant effects. The beneficial role of health insurance was evident only for women, and that of more education only for men. Overall, our CIND results seem rather unstable, consistent also with previous research [35]; CIND is an intermediate or transition stage between normal cognition and dementia. Previous studies using population-based data have reported that CIND is affected by myriad factors [36], and its measurement is a recognized challenge [37]. The MHAS made changes to the cognitive assessment over time, which could potentially influence the assessment of CIND. To minimize the impact of these changes, though, we classified cognitive status using the five original cognitive domains from 2001 that were also included in 2015. Future research ought to use longitudinal data to understand better CIND and its measurement.

Our study confirmed an increase in obesity between 2001 and 2015. As in previous studies [17,38], we found that overweight and obesity were associated with lower odds of CIND and dementia. This result has been interpreted as evidence of a protective effect of higher late-life BMI for dementia as opposed to mid-life obesity [39]. Others have remarked on the importance of BMI changes during the life cycle to assess this association [40,41].

Rural residence and lack of health insurance are well-established sources of health disparities in populations worldwide, particularly in low- and middle-income countries [3]. Our results confirm that these are important risk factors for a higher likelihood of both dementia and CIND. Regarding health insurance, our results showed a beneficial influence of health insurance in 2015 compared to 2001, particularly among women and among those aged 75 and older [14]. Future research should further examine the mechanisms through which the expansion in health insurance over the period could have benefitted the cognitive function of women more than that of men, including the possibility of better treatment and awareness of diseases among women [10].

Our results with Mexican older adults differ from the results reported by others using a comparable period in the United States. Using a similar approach, results from the Health and Retirement Study reported a decrease in the risk of dementia in the United States between 2000 and 2012 [17]. The authors commented that increasing educational attainment and better control of cardiovascular risk factors were associated with a lower risk of dementia over this period. For Mexico, the higher educational attainment we observed for 2015 was still considerably lower than the gains observed for consecutive cohorts of older adults in the United States and other developed countries. As Mexico experienced increasing rates of chronic diseases, a corresponding better control of the conditions was largely absent. Thus, preventing and treating these diseases represents a critical opportunity to reduce the prevalence of dementia, in addition to the educational gains that will continue to prevail in future cohorts entering old age.

We found that being female, older age, no schooling, lack of health insurance coverage, and cardiovascular risk factors were major contributors to increasing an individual's odds of dementia in 2001 and 2015, mirroring what others have reported for other countries [42]. Overall, we interpret our results to indicate that the individual risk of dementia for a person with a given set of traits—age, sex, education, rural/urban residence, cardiovascular risks, health insurance—was higher in 2015 than in 2001. Other factors that were not included in our models may help explain this time trend and could be the subject of future research.

Our study has several limitations. Our cognitive status classification was not based on clinical diagnoses. The classification of cognitive status for individuals who have data collected in population surveys depends on the definitions used and the information captured by the survey instruments. We classified cognitive impairment in self and proxy respondents using two cognitive screening instruments (CCCE and IQCODE), which correctly identify individuals with normal cognitive function and dementia [28,43], while cognitive assessment of those with CIND remains more challenging [37]. Our data also rely upon self-reported measures to determine if participants have any cardiovascular conditions. This approach has the limitation that undiagnosed diseases may be present; the under-reporting of conditions has been described in previous studies [44].

Despite these limitations, we contribute to the conceptual definition of cognitive status using a population-based survey, with our analyses of national samples of older adults in Mexico, using the same cognitive assessments, and including direct and proxy interviews. These efforts represent a significant improvement in our understanding of the dynamics of cognitive aging in Mexico. Future research using additional MHAS data will benefit from our work and continue to add to our knowledge of this crucial public health concern in rapidly aging societies. Policies and programs could focus on the prevention of cardiovascular diseases and their treatment as a direct strategy to reduce the burden of cognitive aging in Mexico, particularly among rural populations.

5. Conclusions

Countries like Mexico with a rapidly aging population may not experience quick increases in dementia prevalence. The trajectory followed will depend on the prevalence of comorbidities, access to health care, and the treatment and management of such conditions, among other factors. Over the 2001 to 2015 period, older age and higher prevalence of cardiovascular risks were evident, concurrent with gains in education and health insurance coverage among older Mexican adults. These risk and beneficial factors likely produced counteracting effects, leading to a slightly higher risk of dementia by 2015.

Supplementary Materials: The following are available online at https://www.mdpi.com/article/10.3390/geriatrics6030063/s1, Table S1: Descriptive statistics of MHAS participants aged 60 and over in the 2001 and 2015 cohorts by cognitive status.

Author Contributions: Conceptualization, S.M.-A., J.A., B.D., M.A.G., A.M.-O., J.L.S., R.S.-T. and R.W.; Formal analysis, S.M.-A., J.A., B.D., M.A.G., A.M.-O., J.L.S., R.S.-T. and R.W.; Methodology, S.M.-A., J.A., B.D., M.A.G., A.M.-O., J.L.S., R.S.-T. and R.W.; Writing—original draft, S.M.-A., J.A., B.D., M.A.G., A.M.-O., J.L.S., R.S.-T. and R.W.; Writing—review & editing, S.M.-A., J.A., B.D., M.A.G., A.M.-O., J.L.S., R.S.-T. and R.W. All authors have read and agreed to the published version of the manuscript.

Funding: The MHAS data is supported by the National Institute on Aging at the National Institutes of Health (grant number R01 AG018016) and the Statistical Bureau in Mexico (Instituto Nacional de Estadística y Geografia, INEGI). This research was supported by the National Institute on Aging at the National Institutes of Health (grant number R00 AG058799 to JS); and by the Nebraska Tobacco Settlement Biomedical Research Development Funds (to MG).

Institutional Review Board Statement: The MHAS protocols and instruments were approved, in the US, by the Institutional Review Board of the University of Texas Medical Branch (IRB Protocol #11-061), and in Mexico, by the National Institute of Statistics (INEGI) and the National Institute of Public Health (INSP). All procedures were done in accord with the Helsinki Declaration of 1975.

Informed Consent Statement: Informed consent was obtained from all subjects involved in the study.

Data Availability Statement: Publicly available datasets were analyzed in this study. This data can be found here: www.MHASweb.org (accessed on 4 December 2020).

Acknowledgments: We acknowledge support from the University of Texas Medical Branch Sealy Center on Aging, and its World Health Organization/Pan American Health Organization Collaborating Center on Aging and Health. These institutions had no role in the analysis or interpretation of the data, writing of the article, or the decision to submit the article for publication.

Conflicts of Interest: The authors declare no conflict of interest.

References

1. Maestre, G.E. Assessing dementia in resource-poor regions. *Curr. Neurol. Neurosci. Rep.* **2012**, *12*, 511–519. [CrossRef] [PubMed]
2. Downer, B.; Veeranki, S.P.; Wong, R. A Late Life Risk Index for Severe Cognitive Impairment in Mexico. *J. Alzheimers Dis.* **2016**, *52*, 191–203. [CrossRef]
3. Saenz, J.L.; Downer, B.; Garcia, M.A.; Wong, R. Cognition and Context: Rural-Urban Differences in Cognitive Aging Among Older Mexican Adults. *J. Aging Health* **2018**, *30*, 965–986. [CrossRef] [PubMed]
4. Rojas-Martinez, R.; Basto-Abreu, A.; Aguilar-Salinas, C.A.; Zarate-Rojas, E.; Villalpando, S.; Barrientos-Gutierrez, T. Prevalence of previously diagnosed diabetes mellitus in Mexico. *Salud Publica Mex.* **2018**, *60*, 224–232. [CrossRef] [PubMed]
5. Campos-Nonato, I.; Hernández-Barrera, L.; Flores-Coria, A.; Gómez-Álvarez, E.; Barquera, S. Prevalencia, diagnóstico y control de hipertensión arterial en adultos mexicanos en condición de vulnerabilidad. Resultados de la Ensanut 100k. *Salud Publica Mex.* **2019**, *61*, 888–897. [CrossRef]
6. Diaz-Venegas, C.; Samper-Ternent, R.; Michaels-Obregon, A.; Wong, R. The effect of educational attainment on cognition of older adults: Results from the Mexican Health and Aging Study 2001 and 2012. *Aging Ment. Health* **2019**, *23*, 1586–1594. [CrossRef] [PubMed]
7. Veeranki, S.P.; Downer, B.; Jupiter, D.; Kuo, Y.F.; Raji, M.; Calhoun, W.; Wong, R. Chronic Respiratory Disease and Cognitive Impairment in Older Mexican Adults. *Neurol. India* **2019**, *67*, 1539. [CrossRef]
8. Avila, J.C.; Mejia Arango, S.; Jupiter, D.; Downer, B.; Wong, R. The effect of diabetes on the cognitive trajectory of older adults in Mexico and the U.S. *J. Gerontol. B Psychol. Sci. Soc. Sci.* **2020**. [CrossRef]
9. Payne, C.F.; Wong, R. Expansion of disability across successive Mexican birth cohorts: A longitudinal modelling analysis of birth cohorts born 10 years apart. *J. Epidemiol. Community Health* **2019**, *73*, 900–905. [CrossRef]
10. Beltrán-Sánchez, H.; Drumond-Andrade, F.C.; Riosmena, F. Contribution of socioeconomic factors and health care access to the awareness and treatment of diabetes and hypertension among older Mexican adults. *Salud Publica Mex.* **2015**, *57*, s6–s14. [CrossRef]

11. Pinto, G.; Beltrán-Sánchez, H. Prospective study of the link between overweight/obesity and diabetes incidence among Mexican older adults: 2001–2012. *Salud Publica Mex.* **2015**, *57*, 15–21. [CrossRef]
12. Parker, S.W.; Pederzini, C. Gender differences in education in Mexico. In *The Economics of Gender in Mexico: Work, Family, State, and Market*; Katz, E., Correia, M.C., Eds.; World Bank: Washington, DC, USA, 2001; pp. 9–45.
13. Wong, R.; Michaels-Obregón, A.; Palloni, A.; Gutiérrez-Robledo, L.M.; González-González, C.; López-Ortega, M.; Téllez-Rojo, M.M.; Mendoza-Alvarado, L.R. Progression of aging in Mexico: The Mexican Health and Aging Study (MHAS) 2012. *Salud Publica Mex.* **2015**, *57* (Suppl. 1), S79–S89. [CrossRef] [PubMed]
14. Wong, R.; Díaz, J.J. Health care utilization among older Mexicans: Health and socioeconomic inequalities. *Salud Publica Mex.* **2007**, *49*, s505–s514. [CrossRef] [PubMed]
15. Satizabal, C.L.; Beiser, A.S.; Chouraki, V.; Chêne, G.; Dufouil, C.; Seshadri, S. Incidence of dementia over three decades in the Framingham Heart Study. *N. Engl. J. Med.* **2016**, *374*, 523–532. [CrossRef] [PubMed]
16. Matthews, F.E.; Arthur, A.; Barnes, L.E.; Bond, J.; Jagger, C.; Robinson, L.; Brayne, C.; Medical Research Council Cognitive Function and Ageing Collaboration. A two-decade comparison of prevalence of dementia in individuals aged 65 years and older from three geographical areas of England: Results of the Cognitive Function and Ageing Study I and II. *Lancet* **2013**, *382*, 1405–1412. [CrossRef]
17. Langa, K.M.; Larson, E.B.; Crimmins, E.M.; Faul, J.D.; Levine, D.A.; Kabeto, M.U.; Weir, D.R. A Comparison of the Prevalence of Dementia in the United States in 2000 and 2012. *JAMA Intern. Med.* **2017**, *177*, 51–58. [CrossRef] [PubMed]
18. Parker, S.W.; Saenz, J.; Wong, R. Health Insurance and the Aging: Evidence From the Seguro Popular Program in Mexico. *Demography* **2018**, *55*, 361–386. [CrossRef] [PubMed]
19. Wong, R.; Michaels-Obregon, A.; Palloni, A. Cohort Profile: The Mexican Health and Aging Study (MHAS). *Int. J. Epidemiol.* **2017**, *46*, e2. [CrossRef] [PubMed]
20. Mexican Health and Aging Study (MHAS). Data Files and Documentation (Public Use): Mexican Health and Aging Study, 2001 & 2015. Available online: www.MHASweb.org (accessed on 4 December 2020).
21. National Research Council. *New Directions in the Sociology of Aging*; The National Academies Press: Washington, DC, USA, 2013. [CrossRef]
22. Baumgart, M.; Snyder, H.M.; Carrillo, M.C.; Fazio, S.; Kim, H.; Johns, H. Summary of the evidence on modifiable risk factors for cognitive decline and dementia: A population-based perspective. *Alzheimers Dement.* **2015**, *11*, 718–726. [CrossRef]
23. Stern, Y. Cognitive reserve in ageing and Alzheimer's disease. *Lancet Neurol.* **2012**, *11*, 1006–1012. [CrossRef]
24. McKhann, G.M.; Knopman, D.S.; Chertkow, H.; Hyman, B.T.; Jack, C.R., Jr.; Kawas, C.H.; Klunk, W.E.; Koroshetz, W.J.; Manly, J.J.; Mayeux, R.; et al. The diagnosis of dementia due to Alzheimer's disease: Recommendations from the National Institute on Aging-Alzheimer's Association workgroups on diagnostic guidelines for Alzheimer's disease. *Alzheimers Dement.* **2011**, *7*, 263–269. [CrossRef]
25. Sperling, R.A.; Aisen, P.S.; Beckett, L.A.; Bennett, D.A.; Craft, S.; Fagan, A.M.; Iwatsubo, T.; Jack, C.R., Jr.; Kaye, J.; Montine, T.J.; et al. Toward defining the preclinical stages of Alzheimer's disease: Recommendations from the National Institute on Aging-Alzheimer's Association workgroups on diagnostic guidelines for Alzheimer's disease. *Alzheimers Dement.* **2011**, *7*, 280–292. [CrossRef] [PubMed]
26. Crimmins, E.M.; Kim, J.K.; Langa, K.M.; Weir, D.R. Assessment of cognition using surveys and neuropsychological assessment: The Health and Retirement Study and the Aging, Demographics, and Memory Study. *J. Gerontol. B Psychol. Sci. Soc. Sci.* **2011**, *66* (Suppl. 1), i162–i171. [CrossRef] [PubMed]
27. Jorm, A.F. The Informant Questionnaire on cognitive decline in the elderly (IQCODE): A review. *Int. Psychogeriatr.* **2004**, *16*, 275–293. [CrossRef]
28. Glosser, G.; Wolfe, N.; Albert, M.L.; Lavine, L.; Steele, J.C.; Calne, D.B.; Schoenberg, B.S. Cross-cultural cognitive examination: Validation of a dementia screening instrument for neuroepidemiological research. *J. Am. Geriatr. Soc.* **1993**, *41*, 931–939. [CrossRef]
29. Mejia-Arango, S.; Wong, R.; Michaels-Obregon, A. Normative and standardized data for cognitive measures in the Mexican Health and Aging Study. *Salud Publica Mex.* **2015**, *57* (Suppl. 1), S90–S96. [CrossRef] [PubMed]
30. Cherbuin, N.; Jorm, A.F. The IQCODE: Using Informant Reports to Assess Cognitive Change in the Clinic and in Older Individuals Living in the Community. *Cogn. Screen. Instrum.* **2017**, 275–295. [CrossRef]
31. Angrisani, M.; Lee, J.; Meijer, E. The gender gap in education and late-life cognition: Evidence from multiple countries and birth cohorts. *J. Econ. Ageing* **2020**, *16*, 100232. [CrossRef]
32. Mejia-Arango, S.; Zuniga-Gil, C. Diabetes mellitus as a risk factor for dementia in the Mexican elder population. *Rev. Neurol.* **2011**, *53*, 397–405. [CrossRef] [PubMed]
33. Seidel, D.; Thyrian, J.R. Burden of caring for people with dementia–comparing family caregivers and professional caregivers. A descriptive study. *J. Multidiscip. Healthcare* **2019**, *12*, 655. [CrossRef]
34. Mijajlović, M.D.; Pavlović, A.; Brainin, M.; Heiss, W.D.; Quinn, T.J.; Ihle-Hansen, H.B.; Hermann, D.M.; Assayag, E.B.; Richard, E.; Thiel, A.; et al. Post-stroke dementia—A comprehensive review. *BMC Med.* **2017**, *15*, 11. [CrossRef]
35. Plassman, B.L.; Langa, K.M.; McCammon, R.J.; Fisher, G.G.; Potter, G.G.; Burke, J.R.; Steffens, D.C.; Foster, N.L.; Giordani, B.; Unverzagt, F.W.; et al. Incidence of dementia and cognitive impairment, not dementia in the United States. *Ann. Neurol.* **2011**, *70*, 418–426. [CrossRef] [PubMed]

36. Fei, M.; Qu, Y.C.; Wang, T.; Yin, J.; Bai, J.X.; Ding, Q.H. Prevalence and distribution of cognitive impairment no dementia (CIND) among the aged population and the analysis of socio-demographic characteristics: The community-based cross-sectional study. *Alzheimer Dis Assoc. Disord.* **2009**, *23*, 130–138. [CrossRef] [PubMed]
37. Plassman, B.L.; Langa, K.M.; Fisher, G.G.; Heeringa, S.G.; Weir, D.R.; Ofstedal, M.B.; Burke, J.R.; Hurd, M.D.; Potter, G.G.; Rodgers, W.L.; et al. Prevalence of cognitive impairment without dementia in the United States. *Ann. Intern. Med.* **2008**, *148*, 427–434. [CrossRef] [PubMed]
38. Atti, A.R.; Palmer, K.; Volpato, S.; Winblad, B.; De Ronchi, D.; Fratiglioni, L. Late-life body mass index and dementia incidence: Nine-year follow-up data from the Kungsholmen Project. *J. Am. Geriatr. Soc.* **2008**, *56*, 111–116. [CrossRef] [PubMed]
39. Anstey, K.; Cherbuin, N.; Budge, M.; Young, J. Body mass index in midlife and late-life as a risk factor for dementia: A meta-analysis of prospective studies. *Obes Rev.* **2011**, *12*, e426–e437. [CrossRef]
40. Tolppanen, A.M.; Ngandu, T.; Kåreholt, I.; Laatikainen, T.; Rusanen, M.; Soininen, H.; Kivipelto, M. Midlife and late-life body mass index and late-life dementia: Results from a prospective population-based cohort. *J. Alzheimers Dis.* **2014**, *38*, 201–209. [CrossRef]
41. Naderali, E.K.; Ratcliffe, S.H.; Dale, M.C. Obesity and Alzheimer's disease: A link between body weight and cognitive function in old age. *Am. J. Alzheimer's Dis. Other Dement.* **2009**, *24*, 445–449. [CrossRef]
42. Livingston, G.; Huntley, J.; Sommerlad, A.; Ames, D.; Ballard, C.; Banerjee, S.; Brayne, C.; Burns, A.; Cohen-Mansfield, J.; Cooper, C.; et al. Dementia prevention, intervention, and care: 2020 report of the Lancet Commission. *Lancet* **2020**, *396*, 413–446. [CrossRef]
43. Jorm, A.F. A short form of the Informant Questionnaire on Cognitive Decline in the Elderly (IQCODE): Development and cross-validation. *Psychol. Med.* **1994**, *24*, 145–153. [CrossRef]
44. Downer, B.; Kumar, A.; Mehta, H.; Al Snih, S.; Wong, R. The effect of undiagnosed diabetes on the association between self-reported diabetes and cognitive impairment among older Mexican adults. *Am. J. Alzheimer's Dis. Other Dement.* **2016**, *31*, 564–569. [CrossRef] [PubMed]

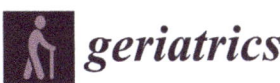

Article

Evaluating the Consistency of Subjective Activity Assessments and Their Relation to Cognition in Older Adults

Cassandra R. Hatt [1,*], Christopher R. Brydges [2], Jacqueline A. Mogle [3], Martin J. Sliwinski [4] and Allison A. M. Bielak [1]

1. Department of Human Development and Family Studies, Colorado State University, Fort Collins, CO 80523, USA; allison.bielak@colostate.edu
2. NIH West Coast Metabolomics Center, UC Davis, Davis, CA 95616, USA; crbrydges@ucdavis.edu
3. College of Nursing, Pennsylvania State University, State College, PA 16801, USA; jam935@psu.edu
4. Prevention Research Center, Pennsylvania State University, State College, PA 16801, USA; mjs56@psu.edu
* Correspondence: Cassandra.R.Hatt@gmail.com; Tel.: +1-316-644-8646

Abstract: (1) Background: Research examining whether activity engagement is related to cognitive functioning in older adults has been limited to using retrospective reports of activity which may be affected by biases. This study compared two measurements (estimated weekly versus reported daily), and whether these activity assessments were related to cognition in older adults; (2) Methods: Participants from US (n = 199) and Australian (n = 170) samples completed a weekly estimate of activity, followed by 7 consecutive days of daily reporting. Differences between weekly estimates and daily reports were found, such that estimations at the weekly level were lower than self-reported daily information. Multivariate multiple regression was used to determine whether total activity, activity domains and the discrepancy between assessment types (i.e., weekly/daily) predicted cognitive performance across three cognitive domains (fluid, verbal, memory); (3) Results: When activity assessments were totaled, neither predicted cognition; however, when activity was grouped by domain (cognitive, social, physical), different domains predicted different cognitive outcomes. Daily reported cognitive activity significantly predicted verbal performance (β = 1.63, p = 0.005), while weekly estimated social activity predicted memory performance (β = −1.81, p = 0.050). Further, while the magnitude of discrepancy in total activity did not significantly predict cognitive performance, domain specific differences did. Differences in physical activity reported across assessments predicted fluid performance (β = −1.16, p = 0.033); (4) Conclusions: The significant discrepancy between the measurement types shows that it is important to recognize potential biases in responding when conducting activity and cognition research.

Keywords: leisure activity engagement; measurement of activity; cognitive performance; aging adults

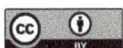

1. Introduction

The "Use it or Lose it" hypothesis of cognitive aging [1], also known as the engagement hypothesis, proposes that more time spent engaging in intellectual, social, and physical activities results in more optimal cognitive outcomes, protects against age-related cognitive decline, and lowers the risk for dementia [2]. Practicing such engagement in leisure activities in older adulthood may therefore buffer the effects of age-related cognitive declines and help promote successful aging. While there is some empirical support for the relation between activity and cognition [3], the evidence is far from conclusive and a number of questions and concerns have yet to be answered surrounding the precise nature of this relationship [4,5]. One issue is the time scale over which activity participation is measured, as studies have shown that information reported over different timeframes relates differently to cognition [6]. Specifically, the present paper examined whether discrepancies existed between subjective activity reports that were based on two different reported time frames: weekly estimated versus daily reported activity. Further, given the focus on the cognitive benefits of activity participation, we evaluated how well activity assessments with different time frames predicted overall cognitive performance, and whether the magnitude of the discrepancies in activity between the two frames was related to cognition.

Activity engagement tends to be evaluated using self-report questionnaires of the frequency of typical activity over a certain time frame such as the past week, month, or year (see [4] for a review). The assessment of self-reported activities generally involves the presentation of a list of activities, and individuals are asked to estimate the number of hours they are engaged in each. The challenge with estimating activity participation is that subjective estimations may not be very accurate. For example, research has documented discrepancies between objective and subjective accounts of physical activity participation [7,8]. In general, participants tended to report less sedentary time than what was recorded using objective accelerometer recordings [7]. Outside of the physical activity literature, whether these discrepancies also exist for other forms of leisure activity, such as those involving social and cognitive engagement, is unknown. Objective accounts of these types of activities cannot be obtained as with physical activity information, and because only subjective reports of activity are available, researchers must assume that the information being collected is accurate. However, it is unclear whether the time frame of such self-reported information results in differences in reported information.

Estimates of activity engagement are susceptible to various inaccuracies and biases, including interpretation of the questionnaire itself. For instance, individuals may by confused by questionnaire phrasing, misunderstand the scope of activities to include in answers, and/or misunderstand the time frame of activities they were supposed to report, leading to struggles in accurately estimating the frequency and duration of their activity engagement [9]. Salthouse, Berish, and Miles (2002) discovered that when participants were asked to estimate the duration of engagement in 22 mental and social activities over the course of a typical week, several individuals reported activity totals of more than 24 h a day, suggesting that estimated accounts of activity information may not represent realistic activity patterns [10].

Even more distant retrospective reports of leisure activity (e.g., over the past two years) may be subject to reduced accuracy in reporting given evidence that episodic memory declines with age [11]. Cognitive biases may influence self-reports or estimates of typical activity. Motivation and the emotional experience associated with specific activities likely also influence the relevance and availability of activity-based memories [12,13]. Further, since perceived meaningfulness of experience impacts participation in activities [14], it is conceivable that this could also impact the accuracy of reported activity information. Activities that older adults are highly motivated to engage in but do not exceed their perceived abilities may be more accurately reported compared to other less motivating activities that are perceived as more difficult or associated with feelings of incompetency [15,16]. Individual differences in the strategic processes employed for emotional attention and memory might further explain why older adults would be expected to have difficulty in accurately remembering non-emotional activity information, especially when estimating over longer periods of time [17].

In contrast to estimating activity participation over longer time intervals, recording activity daily may offer advantages. When activities are written down chronologically shortly after they are undertaken, the tendency to under- or over-report certain activities may be diminished [18]. Daily reports may also be less susceptible to threats of bias and less limited by issues related to retrospective self-reporting [4,5,19,20]. When an individual is asked to remember the activities they engaged in throughout the past day (e.g., 24-h period), this information is easier to retrieve because it was more recently encoded and fresher in their minds [21].

When less time has elapsed between actual participation and activity assessment, there is less opportunity to forget activity related information. This is especially true because different types of activities elicit different emotional responses and these responses can impact what an individual remembers about their day versus what they forgot in terms of the type and frequency of activity engagement [12,15]. We reason that longer recall times may contribute to a greater chance of incomplete, inaccurate, or distorted self-reported activity information. Thus, we adhere to the assumption that activities that are reported over a shorter time frame (i.e., at the daily level) may be less susceptible to error and provide a more realistic depiction of activity engagement. Analogous to this assumption, Almeida (2002) argued that recalling stressors at the daily level produces information that is less affected by memory distortions. As the amount of time between the actual event and requested recall increases, the accuracy of information pertaining to the stressful encounter is reduced [22].

The present study focused on contrasting self-reported activity engagement by older adults across two different assessment periods: estimated weekly versus reported daily. Researchers have relied heavily on the notion that retrospective reports of activity information are accurate and outside of the physical activity literature [7], the phenomenon of discrepancies in reported activity information has never been tested. Samples from two different studies, one conducted in the United States and the other conducted in Australia were used to test the phenomenon of discrepancies in self-reported activity information. Our first aim was to evaluate whether older adults' estimates of typical weekly activity matched the total summation of daily reported activity over a 7-day period. Given the greater likelihood for biases and errors in recall for the activity estimates [10,23,24], we hypothesized that total time spent in activity based on weekly estimates would be significantly higher than the totals of daily activity reports. Second, we examined whether one activity assessment (daily or weekly) was a stronger predictor of cognitive performance. In line with our prior reasoning that a shorter assessment window may provide a less biased report of activity [12,19], we expected daily reports to more strongly correspond to cognitive performance in older adults.

Finally, we were interested in whether cognitive functioning differed for individuals whose weekly and daily assessments were relatively similar, and those who had large discrepancies between their weekly and daily activity totals. Given the aforementioned cognitive biases, and the roles of motivation, attention, and emotional attachment on the ability to accurately recall activity related information [14], individual differences in the ability to accurately recall activity related information may predict cognitive performance. We hypothesized that individuals who have smaller discrepancies between the two activity assessments may be more capable of providing consistent information; these individuals likely have better cognition than others who show greater mismatch between weekly estimates and daily reports of activity. That is, individuals with greater discrepancy between the two activity assessments may have poorer cognitive functioning compared to those individuals who reported more consistently across the two assessment periods.

2. Materials and Methods

Data from two samples, the Activity Characteristics and Cognition (ACC) study [6] and the TRAnsitions In Later Life (TRAILLs) study [25] were used to assess our research questions. Both samples were used to assess the first question investigating differences in self-reported leisure activity information based on the assessment time frame. However, the second and third aims evaluating the link with cognitive performance were only conducted with the ACC sample.

2.1. Participants

2.1.1. ACC Study

Data from 207 community-dwelling adults aged 60–90 years old living in the Fort Collins, Colorado, and surrounding areas was collected. Recruitment began in 2012 and was targeted towards local aging community organizations through flyers, emails, and advertising in newsletters. The following inclusion criteria were applied: They (a) had to be at least 60 years of age, (b) willing to participate in the entire study, (c) have English as their primary language, (d) have no diagnosis of Alzheimer's disease or other forms of dementia, psychotic disorder or personality disorder, (e) could see and hear clearly with corrective aids, and (f) were not full-time caregivers. All participants scored a 26 or higher on the Mini-Mental State Examination [26]. Eight participants were removed from the analyses for missing data (as described below). The remaining $n = 199$ participants ($M_{age} = 70.74$; $SD = 6.79$, 60 men, 139 women) were relatively healthy, rated themselves as having excellent or very good health (70.1%), and were highly educated ($M = 16.40$ years; $SD = 2.54$). Participants had the opportunity to earn up to $60 for completing the study, commensurate with their participation in the various parts of the study. There was limited attrition over the course of this study; only two participants were excluded from the analyses for not answering any days of the activity questionnaire and six individuals were removed for missing five or six days.

2.1.2. TRAILLs Study

This sample consisted of data from 185 Australian adults aged 51–84 years. Participants agreed to participate in the study by accepting an e-mail invitation link that was sent to all members of a local nonprofit organization (National Seniors Australia) in 2010. Of the original sample, fifteen participants were excluded from the present analyses for not completing at least one of the daily activity questionnaires. The remaining $n = 170$ participants ($M_{age} = 61.98$, $SD = 6.17$) comprised the sample used for the present analyses (72 men, 93 women). These individuals were highly educated ($M = 15.40$ years; $SD = 4.00$), and relatively healthy (68.7% rated themselves as in excellent or very good health). Participants were not compensated for their participation in this study.

2.2. Procedure

For both studies, participants completed an estimate of typical weekly activity first, followed by a week of daily reports to recreate two actual activity measurement methods used in studies. This is in contrast to having participants complete a daily report for a week, and then recall their weekly total activity for that same week. This second method would be influenced by daily reminders from the daily reports and would not represent how activity estimates are typically collected in the literature.

2.2.1. ACC Study

Following providing consent for participation, participants completed a baseline assessment that included health, social, cognitive, and activity questionnaires. Baseline sessions typically took two hours to complete and were conducted one-on-one with trained research staff. A typical weekly estimate of activity was completed at baseline. Participants then completed identical activity questions to the weekly estimates every day for the next week (Week 1). Most participants completed the daily activity reports online (69.9%), while others with unreliable access to a computer were provided with a paper version of the activity reports as an alternative. During Week 2, participants completed a different openended activity daily diary (DD) (DD data not reported in the present analyses because the open-ended questions do not easily match the weekly estimate and daily report activities). Half of the sample completed the daily activity reporting as described (i.e., Week 1: daily activity reports; Week 2: DD), but half of the sample completed the open-ended DD in Week 1, followed by the daily reports in their second week. The online version of the daily report activities allowed access only once every 24 h. Individuals who completed the paper version of the assessment completed an honor pledge on days 3 and 6 confirming that they had in fact completed the questionnaire on the appropriate day and were instructed to leave any missed days blank. Participants received a phone call or email on the first day of the daily activity reports recording period and a reminder halfway through the week. See [6] for further detail of the study procedures.

2.2.2. TRAILLs Study

Participants who accepted the email invitation were given instructions linking them to the online survey site. During the first login, participants completed baseline questionnaires containing demographic, psychological, and social measures as well a weekly activity assessment. The week after initial login, individuals were asked to login to the site and complete up to 7 days of daily questionnaires assessing activity engagement. The participants were asked to complete the daily questionnaire sometime after dinner at around the same time each day within 2 weeks of their initial baseline assessment. Participants were asked to try and complete 7 consecutive days of logging in over the assessment period.

2.3. Measures

2.3.1. Activity Questionnaires

ACC Study

Twelve activities from the Activity Characteristics Questionnaire [6] were presented both at the baseline assessment (estimated weekly) and every day for 7 days (reported daily). These 12 items were chosen for their ease of estimation over a typical week, and ease of recall over a day. In the weekly estimate participants were asked, "In a typical week how much time do you spend engaged in the following activities?": (1) Actively watching TV or movies, (2) Reading, (3) Writing, (4) Interacting with close friends, (5) Interacting with people who are not close friends, (6) Meeting new people, (7) Actively listening to information, (8) Attending community events, (9) Going out shopping, (10) Light-intensity activity or exercise, (11) Medium-intensity activity or exercise, and (12) Vigorous-intensity activity or exercise. The following responses were available: no time at all; some time but less than 15 min; 15 to 30 min; 31 min to 1 h; 1 to 2 h; 2 to 4 h; 4 to 8 h; 8 to 12 h; and 12 or more hours. In the daily assessment, participants were instructed to estimate the amount of time they had spent during the previous day (i.e., from midnight to midnight) engaged in the same activities. The same 12 activities listed above were questioned. The responses available for the daily assessment were the same as for the weekly assessment.

For both the weekly estimate and daily reports the same coding scheme was followed: all ordinal responses were recoded into mean hours to create a continuous ratio scale variable. If a participant reported spending no time in an activity this was recoded as 0 h; some time to 15 min was recoded as 0.25 h; 15 to 30 min was recorded as 0.50 h; 31 min to 1 h was recoded as 1 h; 1 to 2 h was recoded as 1.5 h; 2 to 4 h was recoded as 3 h; 4 to 8 h was recoded as 6 h; 8 to 12 h was recoded as 10 h; and more than 12 h was recoded as 12 h. For time frames that were less than 1-h (e.g., some time to 15 min; 15–30 min) responses were recoded as the highest time possible. For all higher time frame options (e.g., 1–2 h; 2–4 h) responses were recorded as the average of that time frame.

For the weekly estimate, the total time across all 12 activity types, and time estimated for each individual activity was calculated. For the daily reports, the reported hours for each activity type were summed across all seven days to give both total time for each individual activity, and a combined weekly total of hours reportedly spent engaged in all 12 types of activities. The percentage of individuals who completed all seven daily questionnaires was high: 95% of participants completed a full week of daily questionnaires; 4% completed six days; and 1% completed five days.

TRAILLs Study

The activity assessment included items adapted from the National Study of Daily Experiences [22] and preliminary versions of the Activity Characteristics Questionnaire [6,25]. At baseline (weekly estimate), participants were asked to estimate the amount of time they spent in a typical week participating in 28 different activities. Only seven of these activities were chosen for the present analyses to provide a close comparison to the types of activities included in the ACC study. The items were: (1) Going out shopping, (2) Vigorous-intensity activity or exercise, (3) Medium-intensity activity or exercise, (4) Light physical activity (5) Watching television, movies, videos, (6) Actively writing, and (7) Actively reading.

For the daily reports, participants were asked to specify the amount of time they had spent engaged in the same 28 different activities as the weekly estimate, but only over the past 24 h. The response scales for both the weekly estimate (i.e., in a typical week) and the daily report (i.e., in the past 24 h) were the same and the following answer options were available: no time at all; between 0 and 15 min; 15 to 30 min; 31 min to 1 h; 1 to 2 h; 2 to 4 h; 4 to 8 h; 8 to 12 h; and 12 or more hours. The same recoding scheme was used for both the weekly estimate and daily report as was used for the ACC study. The weekly estimate total across all seven activity types, and for each individual activity was calculated. For the daily reports, the reported hours for each activity type were summed across all seven days to give a weekly total of hours reportedly spent engaged in each activity, and then combined across all seven types of activities. On average, participants completed 5.4 daily questionnaires, with a wide range in completion (25.3% of the participants completed all seven daily questionnaires, 32.4% completed six days, 17.1% completed five days, 12.4% completed four days, and 12.9% completed three days).

2.3.2. Cognitive Tests
ACC Study

All cognitive testing took place at the baseline testing session. Cognitive measures included: Digit Span (DS) Backward [27], a measure of working memory; the Trail Making Test (TMT) [28], where Part A measures processing speed and Part B taps into executive functioning; the Symbol Digit Modalities Test (SDMT) [29], a measure of processing speed; and Letter sets [30], a measure of reasoning ability. These four cognitive measures formed the Cognitive Fluid factor. The Cognitive Verbal factor included Controlled word associations [30] which assesses verbal fluency, and Vocabulary [30], a measure of verbal knowledge. Additionally, participants completed the Rey Auditory Verbal Learning Test (RAVLT) [31], which measures verbal learning (RAVLT-total trials 1–5), episodic memory (RAVLT-recall List A), and episodic memory-recognition (RAVLT Recognition). These three RAVLT scores formed the Cognitive Memory factor. Factor analysis of these cognitive measures has been documented elsewhere [6]. For each factor, scores on the individual cognitive tests were converted into T scores to allow for comparisons across measures and summed to create the total cognitive factor score (i.e., Fluid, Verbal, Memory). These procedures were specific to the ACC study, as comparable cognitive data from the TRAILLs study was not collected.

2.4. Data Preparation and Statistical Analysis

All data preparation and statistical analyses were performed using SPSS Statistics for Mac version 23. To address missing data in the ACC sample, mean imputation was used. Participants who recorded missing one or two days ($n = 23$) were given their individual mean for each question for the missing day, and those who missed individual questions on certain days also received their individual mean scores. In the TRAILLs sample, there was considerably more missing data, and 73 participants reported missing one or two days. As such we imputed data using the expectation maximization procedure in SPSS. Little's (1988) Missing Completely At Random Test was nonsignificant, $\chi^2(15) = 14.17$, $p = 0.51$ meaning that the data was missing at random.

First, to check that the two measures (weekly estimates and daily reports totaled across the week) in each sample were related, bivariate Pearson's correlations were conducted. Large, significant correlations would imply that the two activity assessments are very closely related to each other, whereas moderate correlations between the two measures would provide support for our argument that the two assessments are related but potentially provide two different types of respondent information, based on the cognitive interferences previously discussed. Next, paired sample t-tests were used to evaluate differences between weekly estimated activity and reported daily activity (summed across 7-days) for both the ACC and TRAILLs data. We analyzed both differences in individual activity questions (across all activity types) and overall weekly activity (summed total across all activity questions). Differences were considered significant at the $p = 0.01$ level. We chose this more conservative significance cut-off to correct for multiple comparisons (i.e., t-tests), but adhered to the 0.05 cutoff for the other analyses described below as the multivariate nature of multivariate multiple regression (MMR) analysis inherently reduces the likelihood of type-1 error.

MMR was then conducted with the ACC data to determine whether either of the activity assessments (weekly or daily) predicted cognitive ability across the three cognitive factors: Fluid, Verbal, Memory. In addition to an MMR with total activity as the primary predictors, we conducted an MMR examining whether different activity domains for each assessment type predicted cognition. Cognitive (reading; writing; listening to new information), social (interacting with close and not close others; meeting new people; community events; shopping), and physical (light, medium, and vigorous intensity exercise) activity domains were created, informed by exploratory factor analyses and theoretical groupings consistent with other literature [6]. The activity of TV and movie watching was excluded from the total activity calculation and the activity domains as this activity has been consistently reported to have a negative association with cognitive ability. In this domain-specific MMR analysis, the three activity domains for the weekly assessment, three activity domains for the daily assessment, and covariates served as predictors of performance across three cognitive outcomes [6].

Finally, a separate MMR analysis was also conducted to determine if the amount of discrepancy between activity assessments (mean difference between weekly and daily activity) was related to performance across the three cognitive domains. In this analysis, difference scores for total activity reported across both weekly and daily assessments was calculated by subtracting the total reported daily activity (across all 7 days) from weekly estimated activity for each participant. An additional MMR analysis examined discrepancy by activity domain, where the difference scores for each of the three activity domains were simultaneously entered into the model predicting cognition.

3. Results

3.1. Differences between Estimated Weekly Activity and Daily Reported Activity

To contrast whether there were differences in the amount of activity hours reported using two different types of activity assessments (weekly versus daily) we conducted paired samples t-tests. Table 1 (ACC) and Table 2 (TRAILLs) provides descriptive statistics for all activities included in both studies.

Table 1. ACC Study: Estimated Weekly and Reported Daily Activity (summed over 1 week) for 12 Activity Items (Hours/Week).

Activity Items	Weekly Estimate M (SD)	Daily Report (Weekly Sum) M (SD)	Mean Difference M (SD)	p
Actively Watching TV/movies	7.76 (4.29)	11.52 (3.56)	−3.77 (4.32)	<0.001
Reading	9.69 (3.21)	12.88 (0.68)	−3.20 (3.17)	<0.001
Writing	4.97 (3.93)	9.96 (4.06)	−4.98 (4.74)	<0.001
Interacting with close friends	7.65 (4.08)	12.37 (2.29)	−4.72 (4.24)	<0.001
Interaction with not close friends	5.37 (3.99)	12.14 (2.20)	−6.77 (4.38)	<0.001
Meeting new people	1.29 (1.86)	5.77 (4.44)	−4.47 (4.46)	<0.001
Actively listening to information	5.89 (3.87)	12.08 (2.53)	−6.18 (4.15)	<0.001
Attending community events	2.66 (2.50)	6.17 (4.91)	−3.52 (4.89)	<0.001
Going out shopping	3.00 (2.43)	9.54 (3.76)	−6.54 (4.11)	<0.001
Light-intensity activity/exercise	5.79 (3.94)	11.49 (3.14)	−5.70 (4.46)	<0.001
Medium-intensity activity/exercise	3.96 (3.11)	8.68 (4.75)	−4.72 (4.77)	<0.001
Vigorous-intensity activity/exercise	2.14 (2.93)	3.80 (4.92)	−1.66 (5.07)	<0.001
Total activity	60.20 (19.91)	116.41 (16.80)	−56.21 (22.97)	<0.001

Note. p values from paired-samples t-tests ($df = 198$ in all cases).

Table 2. TRAILLs Study: Estimated Weekly and Reported Daily Activity (summed over 1 week) for 12 Activity Items (Hours/Week).

Activity Items	Weekly Estimate M (SD)	Daily Report (Weekly Sum) M (SD)	Mean Difference M (SD)	p
TV, Movies, Videos	7.42 (3.71)	15.68 (9.18)	−8.26 (7.82)	<0.001
Actively Reading	5.65 (3.51)	9.17 (6.98)	−3.52 (6.07)	<0.001
Actively Writing	4.54 (3.74)	6.73 (7.42)	−2.19 (6.63)	<0.001
Going out shopping	2.19 (1.81)	4.83 (5.36)	−2.64 (5.37)	<0.001
Light physical activity	3.88 (3.66)	2.97 (4.34)	0.92 (5.19)	0.023
Medium-intensity activity	3.02 (2.89)	5.85 (6.00)	−2.84 (5.83)	<0.001
Vigorous-intensity activity	1.92 (2.57)	3.79 (3.98)	−1.86 (4.27)	<0.001
Total activity	28.62 (11.57)	49.02 (22.48)	−20.40 (20.20)	<0.001

Note. p values from paired-samples t-tests ($df = 169$ in all cases).

3.1.1. ACC

The correlation between estimated weekly activity and total daily reported activity, across all 12 activity types, was small-to-moderate and positive, $r(199) = 0.23$, $p = 0.001$. A paired samples t-test found a significant difference between the total estimated weekly activity (hours/week) and total daily reported activity summed across the week (hours/week), $t(198) = -34.52$, $p < 0.001$, $d = -3.05$. Estimated weekly activity, collapsed across all 12 activity types, ($M = 60.20$, $SD = 19.91$) was lower than the total summation of daily reports across the week ($M = 116.41$, $SD = 16.80$). Table 1 shows that this difference was also apparent across all 12 types of activities, such that there were significant differences between estimated weekly activity and reported daily activity (hours/week) for all 12 activity types (all $ps < 0.001$). For each of the 12 types of activities measured in the ACC study, estimated weekly participation in that activity was significantly lower than the total summation of daily reported participation across the week. Therefore, participants consistently and significantly reported greater time in activity via the daily reports than on the weekly estimates.

3.1.2. TRAILLs

The bivariate correlation between weekly estimated activity and daily reports was positive and moderate-to-large, $r(170) = 0.44$, $p < 0.001$. There was also a significant difference between estimated weekly activity and total reported daily activity (across all seven activity types summed over the week), $t(169) = -13.17$, $p < 0.001$, $d = 1.14$. Consistent with the results for the ACC study, total estimated weekly activity (hours/week) across all seven activities ($M = 28.62$, $SD = 11.57$) was lower than reported summed daily activity over the week ($M = 49.02$, $SD = 22.48$). Table 2 demonstrates that the pattern of mean differences between estimated weekly and reported daily activity over the week was consistent across nearly all the seven activity types (all $p < 0.001$). The exception was light physical activity, $t(169) = 2.30$, $p = 0.02$, $d = 0.23$, which showed participants' weekly estimations ($M = 3.88$, $SD = 3.66$) were greater than their total reported daily activity ($M = 2.97$, $SD = 4.34$); however, this test was not statistically significant based on the cutoff of $p = 0.01$.

3.2. Predictors of Cognitive Performance

Using the ACC data, MMR was performed to examine which activity assessment, weekly or daily, predicted cognitive performance across three dependent variable factors: Fluid, Verbal, and Memory. Total activity for both assessments were entered as independent predictors, and age and years of education were both entered as covariates.

The overall multivariate R^2 effect was significant, $F (12, 505.63) = 6.03$, $p < 0.01$, $R^2 = 0.44$, indicating that the combination of the predictor variables significantly predicted performance on the three cognitive outcomes. Additionally, the predictor variables significantly predicted each cognitive dependent variable, Fluid factor, $F (4, 193) = 9.60$, $p < 0.01$, $R^2 = 0.15$, Verbal factor $F (4, 193) = 7.11$, $p < 0.01$, $R^2 = 0.11$, Memory factor, $F (4, 193) = 7.47$, $p < 0.01$, $R^2 = 0.12$. When examining the parameter estimates however, it appears that these effects were primarily driven by the covariates, age, and education. Neither type of activity assessment total (weekly or daily) significantly predicted cognitive performance, but age and education had significant effects (β coefficients, $p < 0.05$) for Fluid and Verbal cognitive factors; memory factor performance was only significantly predicted by age (see Table 3).

Table 3. Multivariate Multiple Regression Standardized Coefficients for Total Activity, Age, and Education Predicting Cognitive Factors.

Dependent Variables		β	p
Fluid factor [a]	Age	−1.19	<0.001
	Education	1.79	0.003
	Weekly Estimate	−0.00	0.392
	Daily Report	0.08	0.971
Verbal factor [b]	Age	−0.31	0.020
	Education	1.47	<0.001
	Weekly Estimate	0.07	0.180
	Daily Report	0.03	0.649
Memory factor [c]	Age	−1.09	<0.001
	Education	0.30	0.585
	Weekly Estimate	−0.03	0.673
	Daily Report	0.09	0.303

[a] Fluid Factor (Digit Span, TMT Difference, DSST, Letter Sets) $R^2 = 0.149$. [b] Verbal Factor (Controlled Word Association, Vocabulary) $R^2 = 0.110$. [c] Memory Factor (RAVLT Total, Recognition, Recall) $R^2 = 0.116$.

To examine whether activity domains (cognitive, social, physical) differentially predicted cognitive performance, an additional MMR was conducted. Six activity domains (cognitive weekly, social weekly, physical weekly, cognitive daily, social daily, physical daily), plus the covariates age and education served as the independent variables in the model, and the three cognitive factors (Fluid, Verbal, Memory) were entered as dependent outcome variables. Overall, the multivariate R^2 was statistically significant $F (24, 542.96) = 4.13$, $p < 0.01$, $R^2 = 0.42$, indicating that the predictors collectively predicted performance on the set of cognitive outcomes. The multiple R^2s for each of the three dependent variables were also significant, Fluid $F (8, 189) = 5.37$, $p < 0.01$, $R^2 = 0.15$; Verbal $F (8, 189) = 5.30$, $p < 0.01$, $R^2 = 0.15$; Memory $F (8, 189) = 4.80$, $p < 0.01$, $R^2 = 0.13$. Upon examining the parameter estimates, these effects were driven mostly by the covariates, age and education (see Table 4). For the Fluid factor, none of the activity domains across either assessment were significant predictors; however, both age and education predicted performance. For the Verbal factor, in addition to the significant effects of age and education, daily cognitive activity also significantly predicted performance ($\beta = 1.63$, $p = 0.005$). For the Memory factor, performance was significantly predicted by age and weekly social activity ($\beta = -1.81$, $p = 0.050$). Correlation tables between predictor and outcome variables can be found under Supplementary Materials (Table S1).

Table 4. Multivariate Multiple Regression Standardized Coefficients for Weekly and Daily Activity Domains, Age, and Education Predicting Cognitive Factors.

Dependent Variables		β	p
Fluid factor [a]	Age	−1.18	0.000
	Education	1.76	0.004
	Weekly Estimate		
	Cognitive Activity	0.20	0.770
	Social Activity	0.97	0.330
	Physical Activity	−1.27	0.089
	Daily Report		
	Cognitive Activity	0.03	0.973
	Social Activity	−0.33	0.701
	Physical Activity	1.16	0.062
Verbal factor [b]	Age	−0.29	0.028
	Education	1.33	0.000
	Weekly Estimate		
	Cognitive Activity	0.35	0.364
	Social Activity	−0.22	0.694
	Physical Activity	0.57	0.179
	Daily Report		
	Cognitive Activity	1.63	0.005
	Social Activity	−0.75	0.117
	Physical Activity	−0.02	0.946
Memory Factor [c]	Age	−1.07	0.000
	Education	0.19	0.727
	Weekly Estimate		
	Cognitive Activity	1.04	0.095
	Social Activity	−1.81	0.050
	Physical Activity	0.052	0.940
	Daily Report		
	Cognitive Activity	1.00	0.281
	Social Activity	0.69	0.379
	Physical Activity	−0.14	0.799

[a] Fluid Factor (Digit Span, TMT Difference, DSST, Letter Sets). Daily R^2 = 0.149; Weekly R^2 = 0.151. [b] Verbal Factor (Controlled Word Association, Vocabulary). Daily R^2 = 0.147; Weekly R^2 = 0.149. [c] Memory Factor (RAVLT Total, Recognition, Recall). Daily R^2 = 0.125; Weekly R^2 = 0.133.

Next, to examine how differences in estimation reports between total weekly and daily activity predicted cognitive performance another MMR was conducted. The difference score, age, and education served as the independent variables in the model, and the three cognitive factors (Fluid, Verbal, Memory) were entered as dependent variables. The difference score was computed by subtracting the total daily from the total weekly activity (For consistency with prior analyses, we maintained excluding TV in the discrepancy analysis as well. When additional analysis using all 12 activity items, including Watching TV/Movies, was performed the results remained non-significant). All parameter estimates for the total difference score MMR are presented in Table 5. The overall multivariate R^2 was statistically significant, F (9, 467.43) = 7.87, $p < 0.01$, R^2 = 0.54, indicating that age, education, and the amount of difference between activity estimates predicted performance on the set of cognitive outcomes. The multiple R^2s for each of the three dependent variables were also significant, Fluid F (3, 194) = 12.67, $p < 0.01$, R^2 = 0.16; Verbal F (3, 194) = 8.81, $p < 0.01$, R^2 = 0.12; Memory F (3, 194) = 9.89, $p < 0.01$, R^2 = 0.13. However, examination of the parameter estimates revealed that these effects were driven by the covariates, age, and education, as the difference score did not uniquely predict any of the cognitive outcomes ($β$'s were non-significant, $p > 0.05$ see Table 5).

Table 5. Multivariate Multiple Regression Standardized Coefficients of Total Activity Difference Score, Age, and Education Predicting Cognitive Factors.

Dependent Variables		β	p
Fluid factor [a]	Age	−1.22	<0.001
	Education	1.85	0.002
	Total Activity Difference Score	−0.04	0.601
Verbal factor [b]	Age	−0.34	0.009
	Education	1.54	<0.001
	Total Activity Difference Score	0.03	0.494
Memory factor [c]	Age	−1.11	<0.001
	Education	0.35	0.526
	Total Activity Difference Score	−0.06	0.369

[a] Fluid Factor (Digit Span, TMT Difference, DSST, Letter Sets) $R^2 = 0.151$. [b] Verbal Factor (Controlled Word Association, Vocabulary) $R^2 = 0.106$. [c] Memory Factor (RAVLT Total, Recognition, Recall) $R^2 = 0.119$.

In the final MMR analysis, activity domain difference scores were entered simultaneously as predictors of cognitive performance. Overall, the multivariate R^2 was statistically significant $F (15, 524.91) = 5.37, p < 0.01, R^2 = 0.54$, indicating that the predictor variables (age, education, cognitive activity difference, social activity difference, physical activity difference) collectively predicted performance on the set of cognitive outcomes. The multiple R^2s for each of the three dependent variables were also significant, Fluid $F (5, 192) = 8.61, p < 0.01, R^2 = 0.16$; Verbal $F (5, 192) = 5.32, p < 0.01, R^2 = 0.10$; Memory $F (5, 192) = 6.53, p < 0.01, R^2 = 0.12$. Upon examining the parameter estimates, it seemed that the effects were driven mostly by the covariates, age, and education (see Table 6). However, for the Fluid factor there was also a significant predictive effect of physical activity difference scores ($\beta = -1.6, p = .033$). This negative effect indicated that as the amount of estimation error between weekly and daily assessments for physical activity increased, performance on the fluid factor decreased. Correlation tables between predictor and outcome variables used in this analysis can be found under Supplementary Materials (Table S2).

Table 6. Multivariate Multiple Regression Standardized Coefficients for Activity Domain Difference Scores, Age, and Education Predicting Cognitive Factors.

Dependent Variables	Predictors	β	p
Fluid factor [a]	Age	−1.19	0.000
	Education	1.77	0.000
	Cognitive Activity Difference	0.23	0.707
	Social Activity Difference	0.56	0.432
	Physical Activity Difference	−1.16	0.033
Verbal factor [b]	Age	−0.35	0.008
	Education	1.55	0.000
	Cognitive Activity Difference	−0.13	0.719
	Social Activity Difference	0.30	0.478
	Physical Activity Difference	0.15	0.640
Memory Factor [c]	Age	−1.09	0.000
	Education	0.35	0.520
	Cognitive Activity Difference	0.50	0.384
	Social Activity Difference	−1.2	0.059
	Physical Activity Difference	0.06	0.914

[a] Fluid Factor (Digit Span, TMT Difference, DSST, Letter Sets). Daily $R^2 = 0.149$; Weekly $R^2 = 0.162$. [b] Verbal Factor (Controlled Word Association, Vocabulary). Daily $R^2 = 0.147$; Weekly $R^2 = 0.099$. [c] Memory Factor (RAVLT Total, Recognition, Recall). Daily $R^2 = 0.125$; Weekly $R^2 = 0.123$.

4. Discussion

The present study aimed to systematically test for differences between two types of self-reported activity assessments: one that asked for a weekly estimate of activity, and another that asked for daily reports of activity participation. We also investigated whether these activity assessments were predictive of cognitive performance. Our findings showed that differences do indeed exist between activity assessments, where individuals tended to estimate significantly less weekly activity participation compared to when they reported their participation at the end of each day. Importantly, this difference was demonstrated in two different samples of older adults, from different countries. Interestingly, when activity assessments were totaled, neither predicted cognition; however, when activity was grouped by domain (cognitive, social, physical), different domains significantly predicted different cognitive outcomes. Further, while the magnitude of discrepancy in total activity did not significantly predict cognitive performance, domain specific differences did. These differential trends support the notion that using multiple forms of activity assessment may be rewarding for future research.

In our study, both samples displayed significant differences between activity information based on a weekly estimate versus daily reports. A similar pattern of findings emerged across both samples: participants consistently reported less activity at the estimated weekly level than what was reported daily, across almost all activities. The moderate correlations found between the two measures in each sample demonstrate that the two assessments are related but potentially measuring two different constructs. The results show that different types of self-reported activity measurements, conducted over various time intervals, differ greatly in the resulting data. If the amount of activity time being reported is not consistent across days and weeks, then it is challenging to determine which assessments are collecting the most accurate activity information and under what conditions different assessments might be preferred or necessary. There are several reasons why there may have been discrepancies between daily reporting and weekly estimates. This includes that as more time passes between the moment of engagement to when activity is being assessed, cognitive biases become more pronounced and errors become more frequent [14,32,33]. This agrees with other lines of research suggesting that over greater periods of time, motivation and emotional experiences attached to different activities may influence the availability of activity-based memories [23]. Further, it is possible that participants tended to estimate different levels of participation at the weekly level compared to their daily reports as a result of cognitive biases and different heuristics used to recall activity related information [12]. At the same time, an alternative explanation for differences between the activity assessments may be the repeated questioning of activity every day. By completing daily questioning for a week, participants may have increased their awareness of what activities they commonly participated in, leading to reporting a greater number of hours engaged in activity. Further, the order of testing was such that the weekly estimate always preceded the daily reports, so greater awareness of engagement may have also been primed after completing the weekly estimate assessment. Since both daily and weekly assessments were subjective, it is difficult to determine which serves as a better proxy of accurate activity engagement. However, the present research demonstrates that differences are likely depending on time frame of assessment.

The present study also investigated how strongly each type of activity assessment predicted cognitive performance. Given the shorter length of time over which daily assessment occurred and the multiple cognitive, social, and emotional influences that may operate on recalled activity information [14,32,33], we predicted that daily assessments would more strongly predict cognitive performance. Interestingly, total activity for neither assessment type predicted cognition. However, when activity was grouped into cognitive, social, and physical domains, both assessment types predicted different cognitive outcomes. At the daily level, higher cognitive activity predicted higher verbal factor performance, whereas at the weekly level, higher social activity predicted poorer performance on the memory factor. These findings demonstrate that both assessment types have predictive ability for cognition, but the specifics of that relation may differ depending on the nature of the activity. Cross-sectionally, past studies have consistently reported that engagement in cognitively stimulating activities favorably affects cognition. A study by Ferreira et al. demonstrated that activities such as engaging in puzzles was related to better verbal reasoning and working memory [34]. Other cross-sectional studies have also supported the basic premise that increased participation in cognitive, physical, and social leisure activities is related to higher cognitive performance [35–37]. Longitudinally, Ghisletta and colleagues reported more gradual declines in cognitive ability (e.g., perceptual speed) for individuals with higher levels of participation in cognitively stimulating activities such as reading, playing chess, and completing crossword puzzles [38]. While the influence of daily cognitive activity on cognition is in line with what prior research has demonstrated, the negative association between weekly social activity and memory performance was unexpected. Research conducted by Lövden and colleagues reported significant longitudinal associations between participation in social activities (e.g., sport, hobbies, playing games, attending cultural events), and perceptual speed over a six-year period, suggesting a dynamic lead-lag association between activity and cognition [39]. One possible explanation for this inconsistent finding is the potential overlap of functional aspects across different activity domains. For example, attending a community event may involve multiple domains of activity, as it occurs in a social setting, may involve cognitive skill-acquisition (e.g., listening to new information), as well as physical mobility to drive, walk, or bike to the location where the event is being held. This example demonstrates the difficulty with subjective interpretation of activity assessments and emphasizes the need for more research that analyzes the structural associations between different types of activities.

The findings reported here support prior research by Bielak [6] that used the same ACC sample, highlighting different effects on cognition based on the type of activity assessment. Both activity time reported in daily questionnaires and an activity questionnaire that recorded the frequency of participation over the past 2 years predicted unique variability in the cognitive factors. It seems that the specific type of activity scale used, the length of assessment time, and how the questionnaire is administered may all contribute to differences in reported findings.

The total amount of discrepancy between the two activity assessments did not significantly predict cognition, showing that how consistently individuals reported activity time was not related to better cognitive performance. However, when activity domains were used, differences in the physical activity domain predicted fluid factor performance. Greater discrepancy between weekly and daily physical activity predicted poorer fluid performance. This finding supported our hypothesis that individuals with greater differences in estimated activity would have poorer performance; however, this result was specific to physical forms of activity. It is unclear why greater discrepancy in physically specific activities was related to cognitive performance, and particularly only to fluid performance. If the discrepancy in activity reporting was telling of how cognizant a person is of their activity engagement, we would have expected the relation to apply to all three cognitive factors, including memory and fluid ability. This finding speaks to the value of examining activity types individually, collectively, and across different domains.

It is possible that different types of assessments provide different depictions of activity engagement because they are influenced by different underlying constructs. Asking participants to recall typical weekly activity patterns could make them more likely to draw upon self-schemas of what kind of person they believe themselves to be. For example, if a person views themselves as being physically fit and as leading an active and healthy lifestyle, they may be more likely to report that the activities they engage in, at the weekly level, are in line with these perspectives. This is in contrast to asking people to recall their activity over shorter periods of time such as at the daily level, which could allow for individuals to report less biased information about their recent activities without heavily relying on schematics or predispositions of what they typically do and how they perceive themselves [23,40]. This argument is in line with the heuristics and biases approach where people judge the likelihood of an event by the ease for which instances can be recalled [41]. At the daily level, activity reporting would be more consistent with the experienced self, which is present in the moment and representative of what an individual has actually been doing. On the other hand, estimated weekly activity would be more representative of the remembered self, which is influenced by availability and representativeness of what constitutes a "typical" week of activity for that person. These explanations are essential to consider when distinguishing findings from studies that used activity assessments with different time frames.

It is important to acknowledge that while our results were consistent across the two samples, differences between the ACC and TRAILLs studies including compensation, retention, compliance, and how assessment information was collected may have had implications on our findings. However, any impact likely would have been minimal. Differences in compensation between the samples may have impacted participants' motivation to complete all parts of the study; however, attrition rates for both studies were quite low. Methods for retention were also different across the two samples, where email or phone call reminders of the daily questionnaire were provided in the ACC study. In contrast, there were no reminders provided in TRAILLs. The rates of compliance were also very different across studies; while 95% of participants completed a full week of daily questionnaires in the ACC study, only 25.3% of participants in the TRAILLs study completed all seven days of questionnaires. We tested for individual differences (age, gender, education, and self-rated health) associated with compliance rates in each study, but there were no significant differences between individuals who completed all seven days and those who completed less than the full week for either study.

Another difference between studies was the mode (online/paper) for which activity assessments were collected. In the ACC study, all participants completed a paper version of the activity assessment, in person, at the baseline testing session, followed by online daily questionnaires for the majority of the sample (69.9%). Those who did not have reliable access to a computer were provided an alternate paper version of the daily assessment. Differences in the mode of administration (online/paper) was not statistically controlled for in the ACC study but prior statistical models have shown no influence on activity results [6]. In the TRAILLs study, all participants completed both baseline (weekly) and daily assessments online and no paper alternative was offered. Since participants were not given an option for alternative paper testing in TRAILLS, if they did not have access to a computer they could not participate, influencing who participated in the study.

Lastly, the number of activity items included on the questionnaires differed across studies. Twelve activity questions were assessed in ACC versus seven in TRAILLs, and there were slight differences in the phrasing of the questions, including that ACC requested information on activity participation from midnight to midnight of the previous day, versus the past 24 h in TRAILLs. Even with the differences in study design between the two samples, our main finding that daily reports were higher than weekly estimations of activity, was consistent across both samples. Further, the slight variations in protocol in fact demonstrate the reliability of the findings.

One limitation of our study is that both samples consisted of relatively healthy, highly educated individuals, limiting the generalizability of our findings. While samples differed in their geographic location (i.e., United States and Australia), future research is needed using larger, more diverse cohorts. In addition, the study-design was cross-sectional; longitudinal research is warranted to better understand how the relationship between engagement in specific activities relates to cognitive performance across time. Additionally, because we did not have an objective record of activity engagement for each participant, we were unable to conclude that either type of assessment (estimated weekly or reported daily) is a more accurate representation of actual activity patterns in older adults. The issue of needing to identify ideal methods for measuring activity engagement, has been noted by others [4,5]. It may also be reasonable to use a variety of activity assessments, since multiple questionnaires seem to provide different information about activity engagement and how it relates to cognition [6].

To fully understand the relative importance of daily activity participation and its impact on cognitive functioning, more refined measurement tools and shorter data collection periods are suggested. It is advantageous to assess activity engagement multiple times per day, sampling moments in respondent's lives through experience sampling methods [42,43]. The development of ecological momentary assessment (EMA), which captures individuals' momentary responses within their daily lives, has marked a notable advance in the measurement of adult aging across the lifespan, while avoiding the distortions that may affect delayed recall, reducing the accuracy of self-reported information [43,44]. In fact, the best approach may be longitudinal studies that collect daily activity and cognitive information using EMA approaches in addition to longer term-assessments, providing the opportunity to evaluate how the relationship between lifestyle activity engagement and cognition operates at both the daily level and over years. Future studies that incorporate EMA will provide valuable insight into the nature of how the temporal relationship between activity engagement and cognition operates, and under what conditions and contexts activities are most beneficial for improving the daily lives and functioning of older adults.

5. Conclusions

This study compared two types of activity assessments (estimated weekly and reported daily) to evaluate the consistency of the information, and to determine if one was a stronger predictor of cognitive performance. This study is innovative because prior research has had no other choice but to assume that different assessments produce similar and consistent information about activity engagement, which does not seem to be the case. A shorter assessment period (reported daily activity) resulted in significantly greater reported activity time than what was estimated at the weekly level. The significant discrepancy between the measurement types shows that it is important to recognize potential biases in responding when conducting activity and cognition research. We considered daily reports of activity to be less influenced by cognitive bias and forgetting; however, both daily reported and weekly estimated activity domains predicted cognition but differentially, suggesting that each assessment type captured slightly different information [24]. This study is informative for aging research because it provides clear evidence, from two separate samples, that not all types of activity assessments provide similar, and consistent information. It may be advantageous for future research to use multiple types of assessments where activity is measured over different time frames. Multiple contextual, cognitive, and social influences seem to operate on the consistency of self-reported activity information, and our findings that estimated weekly and daily assessments produced inconsistent self-reported information, that differentially impacted cognition, underscore a clear need for measurement improvement and clarification [4].

Supplementary Materials: The following are available online at https://www.mdpi.com/article/10.3390/geriatrics6030074/s1, Table S1: Correlations between Daily and Weekly Activity Domain Assessment Scores, Table S2: Correlations between Total Activity & Domain Differences, and Cognitive Factors.

Author Contributions: Conceptualization, C.R.H. and A.A.M.B.; Data curation, M.J.S., J.A.M. and A.A.M.B.; Formal analysis, C.R.H.; Methodology, C.R.B. and A.A.M.B.; Project administration, J.A.M., M.J.S. and A.A.M.B.; Supervision, A.A.M.B.; Writing—original draft, C.R.H.; Writing—review and editing, C.R.B. and A.A.M.B. All authors have read and agreed to the published version of the manuscript.

Funding: This research received no external funding. The TRAILLs study was sponsored by the Australian Research Council, Grant Number: LP0989584 in partnership with the National Seniors Australia and the Illawarra Retirement Trust. The Australian Research Counsel, Centre of Excellence in Population Ageing Research also sponsored the research conducted at Flinders University, Grant Number: CE10001029.

Institutional Review Board Statement: The data were collected with approval by the Institutional Review Boards at Colorado State University and Flinders University in Adelaide, Australia. The Colorado State IRB approval number was 00000202, protocol: 12-3274H. The TRAILLs project was approved by the Social and Behavioral Research Ethics Committee at Flinders' University/Australian National University (IRB project: 5529; ethics protocol: 2009/041).

Informed Consent Statement: Informed consent was obtained from all subjects involved in the study. Blank copies of the consents forms for both studies were provided to the editor.

Data Availability Statement: Data available upon request from the corresponding author.

Acknowledgments: The authors would like to thank Tim D. Windsor, faculty of Social and Behavioral Sciences at Flinders University for supporting the development of this manuscript and granting access to the TRAILLs dataset.

Conflicts of Interest: The authors declare no conflict of interest.

References

1. Hultsch, D.F.; Hertzog, C.; Small, B.J.; Dixon, R.A. Use it or lose it: Engaged lifestyle as a buffer of cognitive decline in aging? *Psychol. Aging* **1999**, *14*, 245–263. [CrossRef]
2. Wang, J.Y.J.; Zhou, D.H.D.; Li, J.; Zhang, M.; Deng, J.; Tang, M.; Gao, C.; Lian, Y.; Chen, M. Leisure activity and risk of cognitive impairment: The Chongqing aging study. *Neurology* **2006**, *66*, 911–913. [CrossRef] [PubMed]
3. Hertzog, C.; Kramer, A.; Wilson, R.; Lindenberger, U. Enrichment effects on adult cognitive development: Can the functional capacity of older adults be preserved and enhanced? *Psychol. Sci. Public Interest* **2009**, *9*, 1–65. [CrossRef] [PubMed]
4. Bielak, A.A.M. How can we not 'lose it' if we still don't understand how to 'use it'? Unanswered questions about the influence of activity participation on cognitive performance in older age—A mini-review. *Gerontology* **2010**, *56*, 507–519. [CrossRef] [PubMed]
5. Salthouse, T.A. Mental exercise and mental aging: Evaluating the validity of the "use it or lose it" hypothesis. *Perspect. Psychol. Sci.* **2006**, *1*, 68–87. [CrossRef]
6. Bielak, A.A.M. Different perspectives on measuring lifestyle engagement: A comparison of activity measures and their relation with cognitive performance in older adults. *Aging Neuropsychol. Cogn.* **2017**, *24*, 435–452. [CrossRef]
7. Matton, L.; Wijndaele, K.; Duvigneaud, N.; Duquet, W.; Philippaerts, R.; Thomis, M.; Lefevre, J. Reliability and validity of the Flemish Physical Activity Computerized Questionnaire in adults. *Res. Q. Exerc. Sport* **2007**, *78*, 293–306. [CrossRef]
8. Miller, D.I.; Taler, V.; Davidson, P.S.; Messier, C. Measuring the impact of exercise on cognitive aging: Methodological issues. *Neurobiol. Aging* **2012**, *33*, 622.e29–622.e43. [CrossRef] [PubMed]
9. Heesch, K.C.; van Uffelen, J.G.Z.; Hill, R.L.; Brown, W.J. What do IPAQ questions mean to older adults? Lessons from cognitive interviews. *Int. J. Behav. Nutr. Phys. Act.* **2010**, *7*, 1–13. [CrossRef] [PubMed]
10. Salthouse, T.A.; Berish, D.E.; Miles, J.D. The role of cognitive stimulation on the relations between age and cognitive functioning. *Psychol. Aging* **2002**, *17*, 548–557. [CrossRef]
11. Craik, F.I.M. Age related changes in human memory. In *Cognitive Aging*; Park, D., Schwarz, N., Eds.; Psychology Press: Hove, UK, 2000; pp. 75–92.
12. Mather, M.; Carstensen, L. Aging and motivated cognition: The positivity effect in attention and memory. *Trends Cogn. Sci.* **2005**, *9*, 496–502. [CrossRef] [PubMed]
13. Robinson, M.D.; Clore, G.L. Belief and feeling: Evidence for an accessibility model of emotional self-report. *Psychol. Bull.* **2002**, *128*, 934–960. [CrossRef]
14. Parisi, J.M. Engagement in adulthood: Perceptions and participation in daily activities. *Act. Adapt. Aging* **2010**, *34*, 1–16. [CrossRef] [PubMed]
15. Cacioppo, J.T.; Petty, R.E.; Feinsteinm, J.A.; Jarvis, W.B.G. Dispositional differences in cognitive motivation: The life and times of individuals varying in need for cognition. *Psychol. Bull.* **1996**, *119*, 197. [CrossRef]
16. Verplanken, B. Involvement and need for cognition as moderators of beliefs—attitude—intention consistency. *Br. J. Soc. Psychol.* **1989**, *28*, 115–122. [CrossRef]
17. Forstmeier, S.; Maercker, A. Motivational reserve: Lifetime motivational abilities contribute to cognitive and emotional health in old age. *Psychol. Aging* **2008**, *23*, 886–899. [CrossRef]
18. Juster, F.; Stafford, F. Work and Leisure: On the Reporting of Poll Results: Comment. *Public Opin. Q.* **1991**, *55*, 357–359. [CrossRef]
19. Ariel, R.; Price, J.; Hertzog, C. Age-related associative memory deficits in value-based remembering: The contribution of agenda-based regulation and strategy use. *Psychol. Aging* **2015**, *30*, 795–808. [CrossRef]
20. Dudukovic, N.M.; DuBrow, S.; Wagner, A.D. Attention during memory retrieval enhances future remembering. *Mem. Cogn.* **2009**, *37*, 953–961. [CrossRef]
21. Delaney, P.F.; Verkoeijen, P.P.J.L.; Spirgel, A. Chapter 3—Spacing and Testing Effects: A Deeply Critical, Lengthy, and at Times Discursive Review of the Literature. In *Psychology of Learning and Motivation*; Ross, B.H., Ed.; Academic Press: Cambridge, MA, USA, 2010; Volume 53, pp. 63–147.
22. Almeida, D.M.; Wethington, E.; Kessler, R.C. The daily inventory of stressful events. *Assessment* **2002**, *9*, 41–55. [CrossRef]

23. Parisi, J.M.; Stine-Morrow, E.A.L.; Noh, S.R.; Morrow, D.G. Predispositional engagement, activity engagement, and cognition among older adults. *Aging Neuropsychol. Cogn.* **2009**, *16*, 485–504. [CrossRef]
24. Hess, T.M.; Growney, C.M.; O'Brien, E.L.; Neupert, S.D.; Sherwood, A. The role of cognitive costs, attitudes about aging, and intrinsic motivation in predicting engagement in everyday activities. *Psychol. Aging* **2018**, *33*, 953–964. [CrossRef]
25. Curtis, R.G.; Windsor, T.D.; Mogle, J.A.; Bielak, A.A.M. There's more than meets the eye: Complex associations of daily pain, physical symptoms, and self-efficacy with activity in middle and older adulthood. *Gerontology* **2017**, *63*, 157–168. [CrossRef]
26. Folstein, M.F.; Folstein, S.E.; McHugh, P.R. A practical method for grading the cognitive state of patients for the clinician. *J. Psychiatr. Res.* **1975**, *12*, 189–198. [CrossRef]
27. Wechsler, D. *Wechsler Adult Intelligence Scale*, 4th ed.; Pearson: San Antonio, TX, USA, 2008.
28. Reitan, R.M. *Trail Making Test*; Reitan Neuropsychology Laboratory: Tuscon, AZ, USA, 1992.
29. Smith, A. *A Symbol Digit Modalities Test: Manual*; Western Psychological Services: Los Angeles, CA, USA, 1982.
30. Ekstrom, R.B.E.A. *Manual for Kit of Factor-Referenced Cognitive Tests*; Education Testing Service: Princeton, NJ, USA, 1976.
31. Schmidt, M. *Rey Auditory Verbal Learning Test: A Handbook*; Western Psychological Services: Los Angeles, CA, USA, 1996.
32. Hess, T.M.; Smith, B.T.; Sharifian, N. Aging and effort expenditure: The impact of subjective perceptions of task demands. *Psychol. Aging* **2016**, *31*, 653–660. [CrossRef] [PubMed]
33. Szanton, S.L.; Walker, R.K.; Roberts, L.; Thorpe, R.J.; Wolff, J.; Agree, E.; Roth, D.L.; Gitlin, L.N.; Seplaki, C. Older adults' favorite activities are resoundingly active: Findings from the NHATS study. *Geriatr. Nurs.* **2015**, *36*, 131–135. [CrossRef] [PubMed]
34. Ferreira, N.; Owen, A.; Mohan, A.; Corbett, A.; Ballard, C. Associations between cognitively stimulating leisure activities, cognitive function and age-related cognitive decline. *Int. J. Geriatr. Psychiatry* **2015**, *30*, 422–430. [CrossRef]
35. Vance, D.E.; Wadley, V.G.; Ball, K.K.; Roenker, D.L.; Rizzo, M. The effects of physical activity and sedentary behavior on cognitive health in older adults. *J. Aging Phys. Act.* **2005**, *13*, 294–313. [CrossRef]
36. Bugg, J.M.; DeLosh, E.L.; Clegg, B.A. Physical activity moderates time-of-day differences in older adults' working memory performance. *Exp. Aging Res.* **2006**, *32*, 431–446. [CrossRef]
37. Newson, R.S.; Kemps, E.B. The Influence of Physical and Cognitive Activities on Simple and Complex Cognitive Tasks in Older Adults. *Exp. Aging Res.* **2006**, *32*, 341–362. [CrossRef]
38. Ghisletta, P.; Bickel, J.-F.; Lövdén, M. Does activity engagement protect against cognitive decline in old age? Methodological and analytical considerations. *J. Gerontol. Ser. B Psychol. Sci. Soc. Sci.* **2006**, *61*, 253–261. [CrossRef]
39. Lövden, M.; Ghisletta, P.; Lindenberger, U. Social participation attenuates decline in perceptual speed in old and very old age. *Psychol. Aging* **2005**, *20*, 423–434. [CrossRef]
40. Jopp, D.; Hertzog, C. Activities, self-referent memory beliefs, and cognitive performance: Evidence for direct and mediated relations. *Psychol. Aging* **2007**, *22*, 811–825. [CrossRef]
41. Kahneman, D.; Slovic, P.; Tversky, A. *Judgment under Uncertainty: Heuristics and Biases*; Cambridge University Press: Cambridge, UK, 1982. [CrossRef]
42. Timmers, C.; Maeghs, A.; Vestjens, M.; Bonnemayer, C.; Hamers, H.; Blokland, A. Ambulant Cognitive Assessment Using a Smartphone. *Appl. Neuropsychol. Adult* **2014**, *21*, 136–142. [CrossRef]
43. Spooner, D.M.; Pachana, N.A. Ecological validity in neuropsychological assessment: A case for greater consideration in research with neurologically intact populations. *Arch. Clin. Neuropsychol.* **2006**, *21*, 327–337. [CrossRef]
44. Sliwinski, M.J.; Mogle, J.A.; Hyun, J.; Munoz, E.; Smyth, J.M.; Lipton, R.B. Reliability and Validity of Ambulatory Cognitive Assessments. *Assessment* **2016**, *25*, 14–30. [CrossRef] [PubMed]

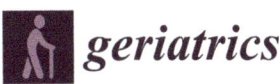

Article

SART and Individual Trial Mistake Thresholds: Predictive Model for Mobility Decline

Rossella Rizzo [1,2,*], Silvin Paul Knight [1,2], James R. C. Davis [1,2], Louise Newman [1,2], Eoin Duggan [1,2], Rose Anne Kenny [1,2,3] and Roman Romero-Ortuno [1,2,3,4]

[1] The Irish Longitudinal Study on Ageing, Trinity College Dublin, D02 R590 Dublin, Ireland; silvin.knight@tcd.ie (S.P.K.); davisj5@tcd.ie (J.R.C.D.); louise.newman@tcd.ie (L.N.); dugganeo@tcd.ie (E.D.); rkenny@tcd.ie (R.A.K.); romeroor@tcd.ie (R.R.-O.)
[2] Discipline of Medical Gerontology, School of Medicine, Trinity College Dublin, D02 PN40 Dublin, Ireland
[3] Mercer's Institute for Successful Ageing, St. James's Hospital, D08 NHY1 Dublin, Ireland
[4] Global Brain Health Institute, Trinity College Dublin, D02 PN40 Dublin, Ireland
* Correspondence: rizzor@tcd.ie

Citation: Rizzo, R.; Knight, S.P.; Davis, J.R.C.; Newman, L.; Duggan, E.; Kenny, R.A.; Romero-Ortuno, R. SART and Individual Trial Mistake Thresholds: Predictive Model for Mobility Decline. *Geriatrics* 2021, 6, 85. https://doi.org/10.3390/geriatrics6030085

Academic Editors: David Facal, Carlos Spuch and Sonia Valladares Rodriguez

Received: 12 August 2021
Accepted: 27 August 2021
Published: 31 August 2021

Publisher's Note: MDPI stays neutral with regard to jurisdictional claims in published maps and institutional affiliations.

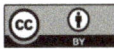

Copyright: © 2021 by the authors. Licensee MDPI, Basel, Switzerland. This article is an open access article distributed under the terms and conditions of the Creative Commons Attribution (CC BY) license (https:// creativecommons.org/licenses/by/ 4.0/).

Abstract: The Sustained Attention to Response Task (SART) has been used to measure neurocognitive functions in older adults. However, simplified average features of this complex dataset may result in loss of primary information and fail to express associations between test performance and clinically meaningful outcomes. Here, we describe a new method to visualise individual trial (raw) information obtained from the SART test, vis-à-vis age, and groups based on mobility status in a large population-based study of ageing in Ireland. A thresholding method, based on the individual trial number of mistakes, was employed to better visualise poorer SART performances, and was statistically validated with binary logistic regression models to predict mobility and cognitive decline after 4 years. Raw SART data were available for 4864 participants aged 50 years and over at baseline. The novel visualisation-derived feature *bad performance*, indicating the number of SART trials with at least 4 mistakes, was the most significant predictor of mobility decline expressed by the transition from Timed Up-and-Go (TUG) < 12 to TUG $\geq$ 12 s (OR = 1.29; 95% CI 1.14–1.46; p < 0.001), and the only significant predictor of new falls (OR = 1.11; 95% CI 1.03–1.21; p = 0.011), in models adjusted for multiple covariates. However, no SART-related variables resulted significant for the risk of cognitive decline, expressed by a decrease of $\geq$2 points in the Mini-Mental State Examination (MMSE) score. This novel multimodal visualisation could help clinicians easily develop clinical hypotheses. A threshold approach to the evaluation of SART performance in older adults may better identify subjects at higher risk of future mobility decline.

Keywords: sustained attention to response task; SART; multimodal visualization; threshold; timed up-and-go; falls; cognition; repeated measures; mobility decline

1. Introduction

Computer-based neurocognitive tests are commonly utilised in research [1], and increasingly, in clinical practice, for both the detection and rehabilitation of cognitive disorders in adults [2]. However, the raw outputs from computer-based tests pose methodological and interpretation challenges, owing to the lack of optimal assays for the precise characterisation of latent neurocognitive processes, and shortcomings of many current methods to allow direct visualisation of multi-modal data that could help clinicians generate more meaningful hypotheses and predictions [3,4]. These challenges are only magnified in the case of computer-based repeated-measures neurocognitive data stemming from large-scale studies.

A common approach in many research designs has been to simplify the raw computer outputs into average features, such as mean and standard deviation of response time, as surrogates of overall performance and variability [5]. However, by simplifying the data in this fashion, much primary information is lost and, consequently, researchers can be left facing unexpected lack of association between results from this approach and clinical outcomes of interest (e.g., disease severity categories). In this scenario, researchers have suspected that the loss of physiologically important information in the simplified data analysis may be responsible for the inability to detect clinically expected associations [5]. Indeed, information averaging can result in loss of power and once a simplified predictor has been created and used in analyses, results should be interpreted considering the dimension of the derived variable, not at the level of the individual original variable [6].

The Sustained Attention to Response Task (SART) is a standard computer-based cognitive test designed to measure the sustained attention, a fundamental executive function for completing tasks that require supervision over time [7]. Sustained attention is a result of the interaction between two different subsystems: vigilance and arousal (alertness) [8,9]. Vigilant attention allows to detect subtle changes in the environment occurring over long periods of time [8,10], and relies on a network of cortical areas including the cingulate gyrus, prefrontal cortex and inferior parietal lobule, as imaging studies have demonstrated [11,12]. The maintenance of an adequate level of arousal is necessary to detect target stimuli [8]. Electrophysiology and functional neuroimaging studies have demonstrated that arousal is activated through a subcortical network including the thalamus and noradrenergic brainstem structures [13,14]. The SART is a continuous performance reaction-time (RT) task designed to promote attention lapses; participants are required to monitor visual displays acknowledging responses for frequent neutral signals (GO trials), but withholding response when detecting rare targets (NO–GO trials) [5,15]. Commission errors (responding to NO–GO trials) or omission errors (failure to respond to GO trials) reflect lack of vigilance, while the RT is a measure of alertness. In older adults, SART has been shown to be correlated with frailty [16] and falls efficacy [17]. However, due to its complex granular intrinsic structure, the optimal way to approach the analysis of SART data remains the subject of debate.

Moreover, recent studies [18,19] have shown a complex network of interactions among different physiological systems and, particularly, between the brain and the locomotor system. We hypothesised that having information on the cognitive and mobility status in the same SART data visualisation would provide clinicians with a more comprehensive framework of general physiological status, even in the absence of clear clinical evidence of mobility or cognitive disorders, and therefore help formulate hypotheses related to potential future health risks.

The Timed Up-and-Go (TUG) is a well-established test to measure mobility and predict risk of falls in older adults [20,21]. In the framework of longitudinal studies of ageing, there is not a unique consensus on the relationship between mobility and cognition. Recent works have shown that baseline quantitative gait parameters are significant predictors of cognitive decline and dementia in older adults [22,23]. However, a previous study in community-dwelling older adults who were cognitively intact at baseline demonstrated the absence of associations between baseline mobility and future cognitive decline, where the latter was expressed by traditionally derived SART variables and other cognitive measures [24].

On the other direction of the association, recent studies have suggested that older participants with poorer choice reaction or stop-signal reaction times may display an accelerated pattern of mobility decline [25] and have a higher risk of incident falls [26]. As this type of study had not previously been attempted with SART data, we were therefore motivated to investigate potential relationships between SART performance and the risk of either a clinically meaningful mobility decline or future falls, utilising novel approaches to classify participants based on their baseline SART performance. Moreover, we considered the Mini-Mental State Examination (MMSE) score as a standard measure of overall cognitive status [27], and in line with previous works, we also investigated the hypothetical association between SART performance and a clinically meaningful decline in MMSE score.

To address the above hypotheses more effectively through the utilisation of the raw SART data, we aimed to devise a new method to visualise the full information obtained from the SART tests performed by a large sample of older participants in a large population-based study, which allowed us to extract features otherwise potentially hidden in derived variables. The individual trial (raw) data visualisation allowed ordering by continuous variables (e.g., age) and also discrete groups of clinical interest (e.g., baseline mobility impairment present versus absent). Furthermore, we formulated a new thresholding method based on the individual trial percentage of mistakes to individuate a subset of participants considered to have a poor SART performance, tested the correlations of this new subdivision with mobility decline measured by TUG and gait speed, risk of future falls, and cognitive decline, and compared its predictive power with other traditional global SART parameters.

2. Materials and Methods

2.1. Dataset

2.1.1. Design and Setting

This research was carried out as part of The Irish Longitudinal Study on Ageing (TILDA), an ongoing nationally representative prospective cohort study of community-dwelling adults. TILDA collects information on the health, economic, and social circumstances of people aged 50 years and over in Ireland. Participants were randomly recruited based on their geographic location. The full design of the study and cohort characteristics have been described elsewhere [28,29]. Wave 1 of the study (baseline) took place between October 2009 and February 2011 and included (i) a comprehensive health assessment conducted at a dedicated health assessment centre (HAC) and (ii) a computer-assisted personal interview (CAPI) in participants' own homes, which involved a collection of detailed data on health, social, and economic factors. Wave 3 of TILDA was conducted between March 2014 and December 2015 (approximately 4 years after wave 1) and comprised the same modes of data collection described above. Ethical approvals for each wave were granted from the Health Sciences Research Ethics Committee at Trinity College Dublin, Dublin, Ireland, and all participants provided written informed consent. All research was performed in accordance with the Declaration of Helsinki.

2.1.2. SART Protocol

The SART is a computerised continuous performance reaction time (RT) task [7]. It requires participants to respond to a repeating stream of consecutive digits 1 to 9 (GO trials) but withhold responding to the digit 3 (NO–GO trials).

In the SART test, each digit appears for 300 milliseconds (ms), with an interval of 800 ms between digits. The cycle of digits 1 to 9 is repeated 23 times, giving a total of 207 trials. The test lasts for approximately 4 min. Participants are instructed to press a keyboard key as soon as possible (with RT automatically recorded using Presentation version 16.5) for each digit presented. RT is null (RT = 0) for the appearance of the digit 3 when no mistakes are committed. For a hypothetical perfect task, there are $8 \times 23 = 184$ non-null values corresponding to the RT when the participant is supposed to press the key, and 23 null values corresponding to the trials when the participant is not supposed to press the key. In practice, over the course of the test, many participants lose attention and commit mistakes. Two types of mistakes can be detected in the data: commission errors (i.e., responding to NO–GO trials), which reflect lapses of sustained attention; and omission errors (i.e., failure to respond to GO trials), reflecting a break from task engagement, also corresponding to lapsing attention [5]. In this work, we considered SART data from wave 1 of TILDA.

2.1.3. Mobility Variables

- *TUG*: TUG measures the time (seconds) taken for a participant to stand up, walk 3 m at normal pace along a line on the floor, turn around, walk back to the chair, and sit down [20]. The test is not just a measure of physical ability, in fact it requires an individual to process instructions, plan and execute movements, focusing on the task and avoiding distractions. This cognitive component makes the test more complex than straight-line walking. Generally, a cut-off of 12 [21,30] or 14 [31,32] seconds (s) is clinically used to discriminate participants with significant mobility impairment. The TUG in wave 1 (TUG_1) and wave 3 (TUG_3) were utilised in this study. Given our aim to capture risk of early mobility decline in this relatively healthy community-based sample, we chose the more restrictive cut-off of 12 s to define clinically significant mobility impairment in both waves. Specifically, we defined mobility decline (*TUG decline*) for a given participant when TUG_1 was less than 12 s ($TUG_1 < 12$) and TUG_3 larger or equal than 12 s ($TUG_3 \geq 12$).

- *Gait speed*: gait speed was assessed using a computerised walkway (4.88 m GAITRite™ (CIR Systems Inc., Franklin, NJ, USA) pressure sensing mat) [24,33]. Participants performed two walks at usual pace, starting and finishing 2.5 m before and 2.0 m after the walkway. The measured gait speed was calculated as an average between the two walks and did not include the acceleration and deceleration phases. Cut-offs between 30 and 120 cm per second (cm/s) are generally used to individuate mobility disability (range 30–100 cm/s) [33] and slow usual pace in older adults (range 80–120 cm/s) [34–36]. We considered the usual gait speed (UGS) at wave 1 (UGS_1) and at wave 3 (UGS_3), and defined *UGS decline* for a given participant when UGS_1 was greater or equal than 100 cm/s ($UGS_1 \geq 100$cm/s) and UGS_3 smaller than 100 cm/s ($UGS_3 < 100$cm/s).

- *Falls*: as part of the CAPI, participants were asked whether they had falls in the year prior to the interview. We recorded the number of recalled falls in wave 1 ($falls_1$) and wave 3 ($falls_3$), and defined as *new fallers* those participants who had at least 1 fall in the year prior to the examination at wave 3 ($falls_3 > 0$) and no falls in the year prior to the examination at wave 1 ($falls_1 = 0$).

2.1.4. MMSE

Global cognitive function was assessed using the Mini-Mental State Examination (MMSE) test, giving participants a score from 0 (minimum) to 30 (maximum) [27,37,38]. We considered the MMSE score in wave 1 ($MMSE_1$) and wave 3 ($MMSE_3$) and, in line with previous recommendations [39], defined as clinically meaningful cognitive decline a decrease of at least 2 points between wave 1 and 3 ($MMSE_1 - MMSE_3 \geq 2$).

2.1.5. Covariates

Several potentially relevant covariates at wave 1 were considered in this work: (a) features extracted from the SART multimodal visualisation (see below), in addition to the traditional SART mean and standard deviation (SD) of RTs (across all trials) both measured in milliseconds (ms); (b) sociodemographic variables: age, sex, and education level (categorised as primary/none, secondary or third/higher); (c) variables expressing the psychological status of participants: anxiety, assessed with the anxiety subscale of the Hospital Anxiety and Depression Scale (HADS-A) [40], which ranges in scores from 0 to 21 (higher scores indicating more symptoms of anxiety); depression, assessed with the Centre for Epidemiological Studies Depression (CES-D) scale [41], which ranges in scores from 0 to 60 (higher scores indicating worse depressive status); and (d) variables related to the physical status of participants: whether or not they were taking any antihypertensive medications (coded using the Anatomical Therapeutic Chemical Classification (ATC) [42]: antihypertensive medications (ATC C02), diuretics (ATC C03), β-blockers (ATC C07), calcium channel blockers (ATC C08), and renin-angiotensin system agents (ATC C09)), had history of diabetes, self-reported smoking (categorised as never, past, or current) and alcohol consumption habits (the answer to the question "Do you have a drinking problem?" (yes, no, or I don't know) was recorded), UGS at baseline, and physical activity status based on the International Physical Activity Questionnaire (IPAQ) (short form) scoring protocol [43] (categorised as low, medium, or high).

2.2. Multimodal Visualisation

All analyses and graphical representations were created with MATLAB (R2020b, The MathWorks, Inc., Natick, MA, USA).

2.2.1. Entire Sample

1. *SART RT representation*: we considered the number of mistakes (commission and/or omission errors) committed within each trial, and the average RT for all correct actions in that trial. We then represented a spot for each trial and participant, the position of which depended on its average RT, and the size on the percentage of errors committed in the corresponding trial. Thus, each participant had 23 spots arranged on the same vertical line, corresponding to the 23 SART trials. SART performance is known to be influenced by age [44]; therefore, we recorded the age of participants and ordered the visualisations by increasing age as a continuous variable. The spots corresponding to different participants were organised horizontally from youngest (left) to oldest (right). For ease of interpretation, ticks were created to indicate a 5-year age change: the distances on the horizontal axis between two consecutive ticks, corresponding to a 5-year range, were not always the same, since most of the cohort was between 50 and 65 years old. Of note, trials where the participant did not press the key at any time and/or some RT were missing, did not have the corresponding computed average RT, and were not plotted in the graph. Bigger spots correspond to trials with higher number of mistakes. Moreover, the spots were also colour-coded based on the percentage of mistakes, going from light brown (0 mistakes) to black for the maximum number of mistakes (8 mistakes in order to have at least 1 RT and assign the position to the spot). Spots with size larger than 2 SD from the mean size calculated across all trials and all participants (excluding missing data and trials with 0 correct actions) were highlighted by white edges in the graph and labelled as "big spots". A complete mathematical explanation of the SART RT representation is given in an appendix to this work (Appendix A).
2. *SART mistakes line*: to further visualise our dataset, we calculated the sum of mistakes made by each participant across all trials, and we represented this value as an additional line function in the same graph above the previously explained cloud plot. The mistakes line function is not linearly related to the size of the spots and indicates a global parameter for each participant over the whole task.
3. *MMSE and TUG lines*: additionally, the graph was enriched by the presentation of participants' MMSE score and TUG at wave 1. These values were multiplied by a factor 3 to be visible at the same graph scale.

2.2.2. Thresholded Multimodal Visualisation

To ease the visual detection of "big spots" and highlight poor performances that may have been 'buried' in the dense cloud plot, a second graph was created containing only the "big spots". All of the above-mentioned notations regarding the coordinates, size and colour of the spots still apply. The curves representing the number of mistakes, MMSE score, and TUG were now limited to only subjects who had at least one big spot.

2.2.3. Application to Categories Stratification and Threshold

We applied the above-described multimodal visualisation methods to allow additional categorisation to discern participants with $TUG_1 \geq 12$ s. Specifically, SART trials for participants with low TUG were presented with dark blue spots, and the trials for participants with high TUG with light blue spots on the right part of the graph, sequentially after the low TUG participants along the horizontal axis. Notably, we ordered participants by age within each category. Therefore, we could appreciate in the same graph multiple levels of information of the dataset analysed: (1) SART RT characteristics across different trials for each participant, and across different participants; (2) distribution of the SART RT by age and for different baseline TUG categories; and (3) global parameters like number of total mistakes, MMSE score, and TUG represented as continuous curves in the top part of the graph (where void spots in the curves were due to missing data for some participants).

2.2.4. Feature Extraction

We extracted some features directly from the multimodal visualisation: (a) mean RT and SD RT, (b) whether or not a participant had bad performances ("big spots"), especially in the thresholded visualisation, and (c) based on the size and colour of the spots, it was possible to understand how each participant performed in each trial, and if their performances were consistent to each other in the whole task in terms of mistakes committed, or if the variation of performance between different trials was high. We subsequently created a new variable that indicated the number of bad performances for each participant (i.e., number of big spots).

2.3. Statistical Analysis

We considered the evolution of mobility variables over time. Specifically, we compared the distribution of TUG and UGS values in the same group of participants at wave 1 and wave 3 using the Wilcoxon test, a nonparametric test used to compare related samples [45,46]. We then compared the TUG and UGS change between participants who at wave 1 did not have any SART bad performances, and those who had at least one bad performance. We compared these two subsets of participants using the Mann–Whitney U test, a nonparametric test used to compare independent samples [47,48]. All the statistical tests were performed in IBM SPSS Statistics version 27 (IBM Corp., Armonk, NY, USA). Statistical significance was set at $p < 0.05$ throughout.

2.3.1. Binary Logistic Regression

Binary logistic regression models were used to predict the binary outcomes that we considered to be clinically meaningful. Specifically, we tested whether the new variable reporting the number of "bad performances" in SART at wave 1 was a good predictor of mobility decline: we assigned 1 to participants with *TUG decline* as defined in Section 2.1.3, and 0 otherwise; correspondingly we assigned 1 to participants with *UGS decline* as defined in Section 2.1.3, and 0 otherwise. Similarly, we assigned 1 to *new fallers*, as defined in Section 2.1.3, and 0 otherwise. Moreover, we also tested the prediction strength of the new variable for cognitive decline, as defined in Section 2.1.4. These 4 dichotomous variables were set as outcomes in the binary logistic regression models, from which we reported the odds ratio (OR) with corresponding 95% confidence interval (C.I.) and *p*-value for each independent variable in the model. The OR expresses the odds that an outcome will occur in the presence of an independent variable, compared to the odds that the outcome will occur in the absence of that variable, therefore if $OR > 1$ the independent variable influences positively the odds of the outcome, if $OR < 1$ the independent variable influences negatively the odds of the outcome, i.e., it is "protective" against the outcome, and if $OR = 1$ the independent variable does not influence the outcome [49,50]. For each binary outcome, wave 1 covariates were used in four different regression models to incrementally determine the robustness of the predictor, as follows: model 1, with just the predictor; model 2, which was model 1 additionally adjusted with mean RT and SD RT; model 3, which was model 2 with the addition of age, sex, and education level; and model 4, which was the fully adjusted regression model, considering also all the other covariates mentioned in Section 2.1.5 (anxiety, depression, hypertensives, diabetes, smoking, alcohol, and IPAQ).

2.3.2. Comparison with Two Other Potential Predictors

In order to test the prediction strength of our new SART feature of interest (i.e., 'number of bad performances') for the four binary outcomes of clinical interest, the same four different binary logistic regression models were applied considering the same covariates mentioned before but substituting the 'number of bad performances' with the global variable 'number of total mistakes' in the whole SART task, and the 'number of mistakes in good performances'. The latter was obtained summing up the number of mistakes in performances that did not reach the threshold defined in Section 2.2.1, and therefore did not amount to "big spots". Of note, every time that we applied the binary logistic regression model (whether adjusted by covariates or not) we considered only one of these three potential predictors, because we were interested to individuate a variable that had good predictive power for the outcome and could be used independently from the other predictors. Indeed, the presence of different predictors would lead to a mixed effect on the outcome probability, and the predictive power would depend on the combination of predictors, and not on the individual predictors. Each adjusted model, considering the three different predictors separately, had been tested for multi-collinearity (based on Spearman's correlation). We compared the OR of the three predictors, whilst noting the degree of overlap in the 95% C.I.s and the corresponding p-values.

2.3.3. Sensitivity Analysis

In order to test the robustness of the new variable *bad performances*, and to evaluate its ability to predict the outcomes in the binary logistic regression models compared to the performance of the other two SART-related predictors, we considered a further logistic model, model 4a, which was model 4 adjusted with a mobility-related covariate UGS at baseline wave 1. In this case, we considered the significance of the three main potential predictors, and compared their OR, whilst noting the degree of overlap in the 95% C.I.s.

3. Results

In total, 8175 participants over the age of 50 years were included in wave 1 of TILDA, of which 5035 attended the health centre assessment. Among those, SART data were available for 4864 participants (54.6% female, aged 50 to 93 years, with mean 61.7 ± 8.3 years). Table 1 presents descriptive statistics for the variables used in this work for the baseline wave 1 cohort ($N = 4864$), and the merged cohort for waves 1 and 3 ($N = 3890$).

3.1. Information Provided by the Multimodal Visualisation

Figure 1 shows the multimodal visualizations based on $N = 4864$ participants. There were in total 1222 "big spots" representing bad performances for 565 different subjects (11.6% of the sample). Among those aged 50–64, 8.2% had bad performances; among those aged 65–74, 17.9% had bad performances; and among those aged 75 years and older, 33.7% had bad performances. In this dataset, the "big spot" (bad performance) threshold, as defined in Section 2.2.1, was 4 mistakes out of 9 for each individual trial. The density distribution of big spots can be better appreciated in Figure 1b.

From $N = 4864$, 4834 had baseline TUG information (data for this variable was missing for 30 participants, i.e., 0.6% of the entire sample); among these, 237 participants had $TUG_1 \geq 12$ s. Figure 2 shows the multimodal visualisation discriminating participants with low TUG_1 from those with high TUG_1. Moreover, within each category, the subjects are age-sorted in ascending order. Considering the participants with bad performances, we registered that 29.1% of participants with $TUG_1 \geq 12$ s had at least 1 SART bad performance, while only 10.8% of participants with $TUG_1 < 12$ s had SART bad performances.

Regarding missing data, in both visualisations there were 83 subjects whose corresponding spots could not be depicted in the graphs. Among those, 20 subjects had 1 or 2 trials where they did not press the key at all having not even 1 RT in that trial. In the rest, there was missing data just for some RT; because of this, it was not possible to calculate the average RT for that trial, and the corresponding spot in the graph could not be created.

Table 1. Descriptive statistics for the whole set of variables considered in this study at wave 1 for the entire dataset (cohort 1, $N = 4864$) and the merged dataset (cohort 2, $N = 3890$). The first part of the table gives minimum and maximum values, and mean and SD for each continuous variable. The second part shows ordinal or nominal variables and their frequency in percentage.

Continuous Variable	Cohort 1 (Wave 1): Mean (SD); Range	Cohort 2 (Merged Wave 1–3): Mean (SD); Range
SART bad performances	0.3 (1.1); 0–21	0.2 (1.0); 0–20
SART: Total mistakes	11.0 (12.3); 0–117	10.3 (11.7); 0–117
SART: Mistakes in good performances	9.8 (9.6); 0–60	9.3 (9.1); 0–60
SART: Mean RT (ms)	385.3 (96.1); 168.9–836.5	383.3 (94.4); 168.9–836.5
SART: SD RT (ms)	72.9 (41.6); 12.8–364.2	71.3 (40.6); 12.8–364.2
TUG (s)	8.6 (2.1); 4.3–39.3	8.5 (1.9); 4.8–28.7
UGS (cm/s)	136.0 (20.5); 28.7–213.9	136.6 (19.7); 43.1–207.5
Falls	0.4 (1.7); 0–52	0.4 (1.4); 0–50
MMSE	28.7 (1.8); 0–30	28.8 (1.8); 0–30
Age (years)	61.7 (8.3); 50–93	61.5 (8.1); 50–90
Anxiety	5.4 (3.6); 0–20	5.4 (3.5); 0–20
Depression	5.6 (6.9); 0–53	5.4 (6.8); 0–53
Ordinal/Nominal Variable	**Cohort 1 (Wave 1) Frequency (%)**	**Cohort 2 (Merged Wave 1–3) Frequency (%)**
Female	54.6	54.6
Education level - primary/none - secondary - third/higher	 21.2 41.9 36.9	 19.5 41.5 38.9
Antihypertensives	13.3	32.4
Diabetes	6.2	6.1
Smoker - never - past - current	 45.9 39.3 14.9	 46.7 39.6 13.6
Drinking problem	12.8(9.1 *)	13.2(7.6 *)
IPAQ - low - medium - high	 27.5 35.9 35.7	 26.9 36.0 36.2

* Dummy group of participants who answered "Don't know" to the question "Do you have a drinking problem?".

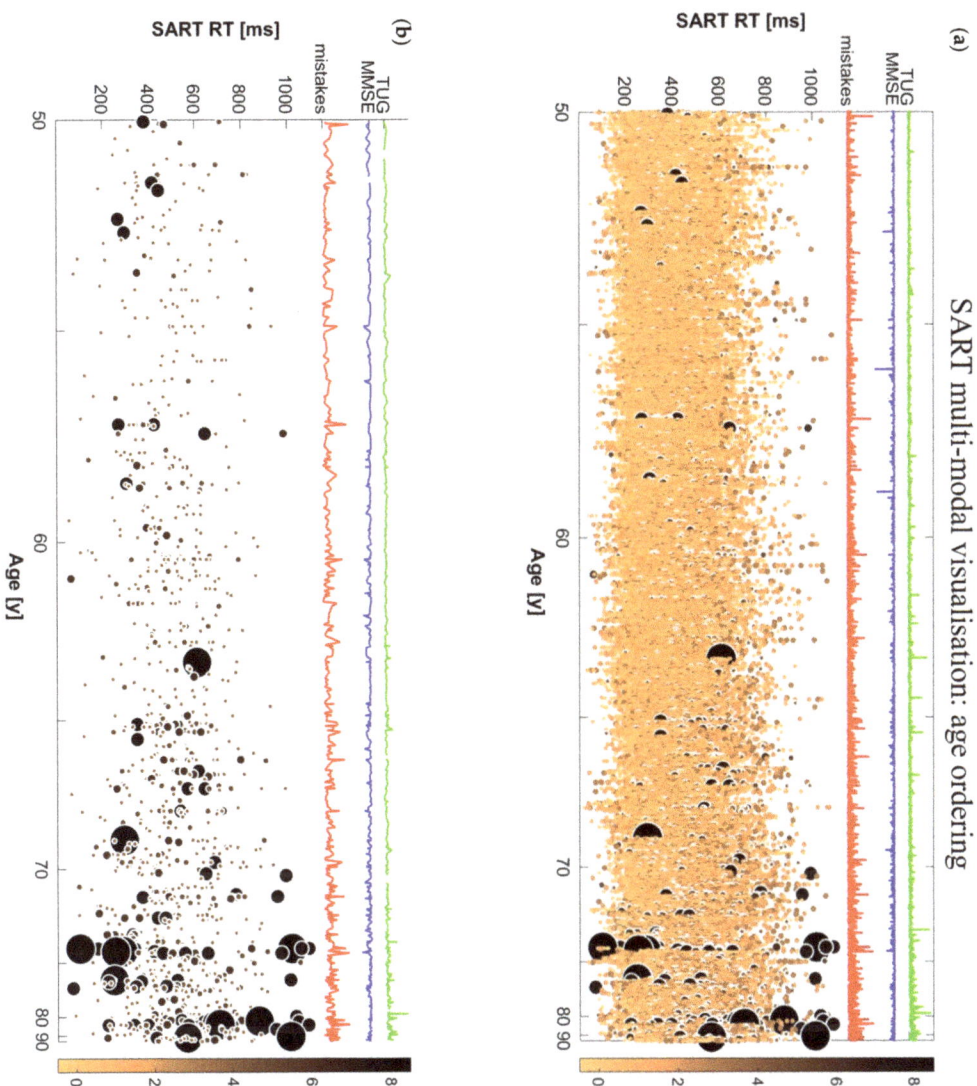

Figure 1. Multimodal visualisation of SART data, (**a**) ordered by age and (**b**) ordered by age with thresholding applied.

3.2. Longitudinal Analysis

The merged longitudinal sample examined at both waves 1 and 3 was constituted by $N = 3890$ participants (54.6% female, ages 50 to 90 years, with mean 61.5 ± 8.1 years). Table 1 shows additional characteristics of this sample. We compared the distributions of *TUG*, *UGS* and *previous falls* at waves 1 and 3, and the Wilcoxon rank sum test suggested that the distributions of the three variables were significantly different: $p < 0.001$ for *TUG* and *UGS*, and $p = 0.015$ for *falls*.

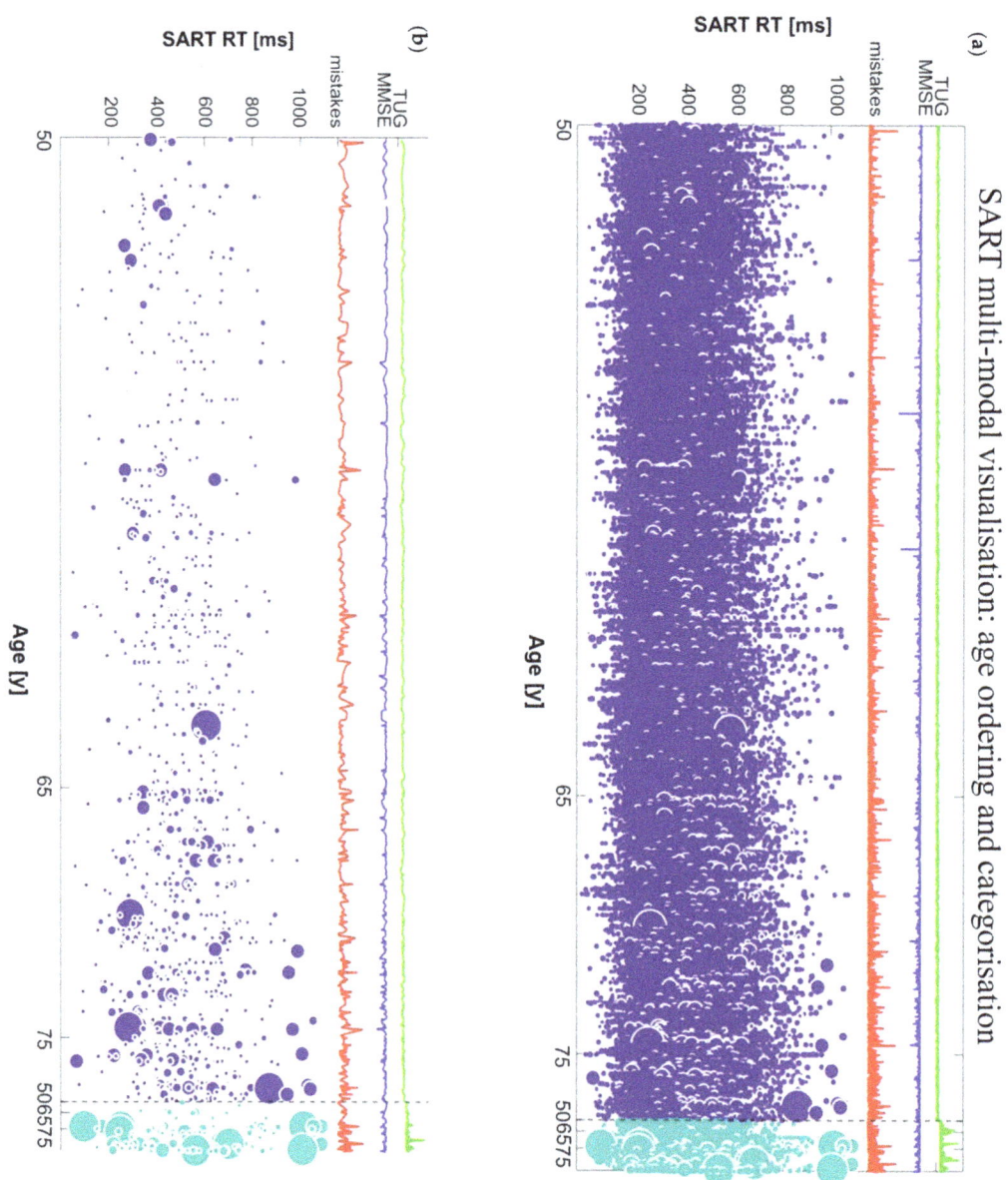

Figure 2. Multimodal visualisation of SART data, (**a**) ordered by age within baseline TUG categories and (**b**) ordered by age within TUG categories with thresholding applied. Dark blue spots indicate participants with $TUG_1 < 12$ s, light blue spots indicate participants with $TUG_1 \geq 12$ s.

Figure 3 shows the mean TUG at wave 1 and 3 for two subgroups of participants: one where participants only had good performances in SART at wave 1, and another where participants had at least one bad performance. From Figure 3, we noticed two elements: (i) TUG generally increased from wave 1 to wave 3; and (ii) the increment of TUG between the two waves seemed more pronounced in participants who had at least one SART bad performance at wave 1. Indeed, the slope of the TUG increment for participants with only good performances was m = 0.871, while the slope for participants with at least one SART bad performance was m = 1.512. The distributions of values for $TUG_3 - TUG_1$ were statistically significantly different between the two subgroups (Mann–Whitney U test $p < 0.001$).

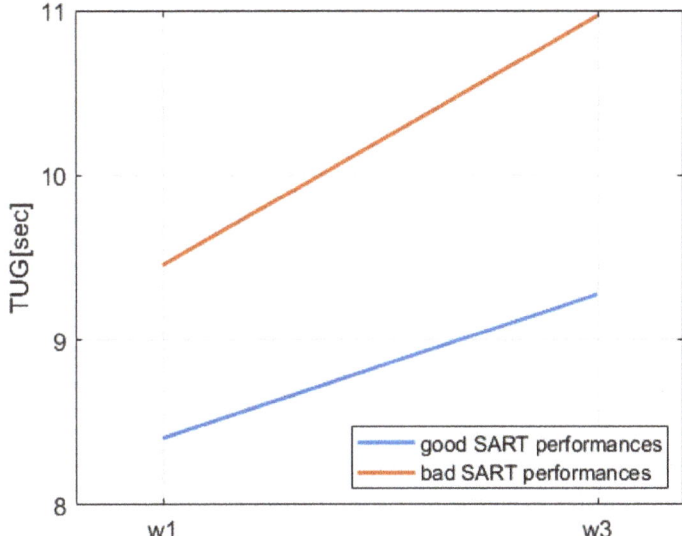

Figure 3. TUG at wave 1 and wave 3 for participants who only had good performances in SART at wave 1 and those who had at least 1 bad performance.

Furthermore, significant differences were also found between the distributions of values for $UGS_1 - UGS_3$ and the number of previous falls at wave 3 for participants with only good SART performances at wave 1 and participants with at least 1 bad performance (Mann–Whitney U test $p = 0.014$ for UGS decrease and $p = 0.016$ for falls).

3.3. Number of Bad Performances as Predictor of Mobility Decline

The three potential SART predictors, *bad performances*, *total mistakes* and *mistakes in good performances*, failed the Kolmogorov–Smirnov and Shapiro–Wilk normality tests ($p < 0.001$, i.e., their distributions were not significantly similar to the normal distribution). We also noted that the standardised residuals were not normally distributed. Therefore, we excluded the linear regression model and any other parametric tests and applied binary logistic regression models for the prediction of the four dichotomous outcomes of clinical interest. In every model, the independent variables passed the multi-collinearity test (Spearman's correlation coefficient $|\rho| \leq 0.422$ for all pairs) and satisfied all other logistic regression assumptions.

As Table 2 shows, the binary logistic regression models demonstrated that the number of bad performances was a significant independent predictor of *TUG decline* ($p < 0.001$ in all four models, OR = 1.287, 95% C.I. = (1.137; 1.456) in the fully adjusted model (model 4), i.e., for every one-unit increase in *bad performances* we would expect an increase of 0.287 in the odds of *TUG decline*, and OR = 1.305, 95% C.I. = (1.130; 1.508) in model 4a). Table A1 in Appendix A shows the results of the fully adjusted binary logistic regression model 4 where the OR, 95% C.I. for OR and p-value for each independent variable in the model are reported. Of note, other significant predictors of *TUG decline* in model 4 were age, being on antihypertensives, history of diabetes, and active smoking status. A high level of self-reported physical activity was significantly protective against *TUG decline*, i.e., those who were highly physically active were less likely to have a $TUG \geq 12$ s after 4 years.

We observe that in model 4a, where UGS at baseline was also considered as a covariate, the variable *bad performances* maintained its statistical significance, while other covariates, which were significant predictors in the previous model 4, lost it (Table A2 in Appendix A). In this case the only significant predictors were the number of bad performances, age and UGS at baseline. Moreover, comparing the OR of *bad performances* across different models applied, we noted that it was stronger in model 1, it decreased in models 2 and 3, and it increased again in model 4, and even more in model 4a, having a difference of just 0.083 compared to model 1.

Table 2. Comparison of the OR and corresponding 95% C.I. of *bad performances*, *total mistakes*, and *mistakes in good performances* for the prediction of *TUG decline* in the binary logistic regression models.

	TUG Decline								
	Bad Performances			Total Mistakes			Mistakes in Good Performances		
	OR	95% C.I.	p	OR	95% C.I.	p	OR	95% C.I.	p
Model 1	1.388	1.256–1.533	<0.001	1.048	1.039–1.056	<0.001	1.060	1.049–1.072	<0.001
Model 2	1.247	1.127–1.379	<0.001	1.042	1.030–1.053	<0.001	1.054	1.038–1.069	<0.001
Model 3	1.207	1.081–1.388	<0.001	1.027	1.015–1.040	<0.001	1.029	1.012–1.046	<0.001
Model 4	1.287	1.137–1.456	<0.001	1.029	1.015–1.043	<0.001	1.026	1.008–1.045	0.005
Model 4a	1.305	1.130–1.508	<0.001	1.030	1.015–1.047	<0.001	1.027	1.007–1.047	0.008

Models for each main predictor, i.e., *bad performances*, *total mistakes*, or *mistakes in good performances*: model 1, with just the main predictor; model 2, adjusted with mean RT and SD RT; model 3, which was model 2 with the addition of age, sex, and education level; model 4, the fully adjusted regression model, considering also the other covariates mentioned in Section 2.1.5 (anxiety, depression, hypertensives, diabetes, smoking, alcohol, and IPAQ); and model 4a, which was model 4 adjusted by UGS at baseline (wave 1). The odds ratio (OR) and corresponding 95% confidence interval (C.I.) give a measure of the influence of the predictor on the outcome; the *p*-value expresses the statistical significance of the predictor in the model.

The variable *bad performances* was a significant predictor for *UGS decline* only in model 1 ($p < 0.001$, OR = 1.232, 95% C.I. = (1.102; 1.377)), namely without considering other covariates. In models 2, 3, and 4, the number of bad performances was not a significant predictor ($p > 0.05$). Table A3 in Appendix A shows the results of the fully adjusted model 4 where the OR, 95% C.I. for OR, and *p*-value for each independent variable in the model are reported. In this case the only significant independent predictors were age and being on antihypertensive medications.

Furthermore, we applied the same binary logistic regression models for the prediction of becoming a new faller. As shown in Table 3, in models 1, 2, 4, and 4a the *bad performances* feature resulted a significant predictor ($p < 0.021$ in the four models, OR = 1.114, 95% C.I. = (1.026; 1.211) in the fully adjusted Model 4, and OR = 1.110, 95% C.I. = (1.021; 1.207) in model 4a), while in model 3 its *p*-value was borderline ($p = 0.057$), having the absolute value of the difference from the significance threshold $\alpha = 0.05$ smaller than 10^{-2} ($|p - \alpha| < 0.01$). Table A4 in Appendix A shows the results of the fully adjusted binary logistic regression model 4 reporting the OR, 95% C.I. for OR and *p*-value for each independent variable. Of note, the only other significant predictor of becoming a new faller was age ($p = 0.004$, OR = 1.020, 95% C.I. = (1.006; 1.034)). Table A5 in Appendix A presents similar results for model 4a: again the only other significant predictor of becoming a new faller was age ($p = 0.011$, OR = 1.019, 95% C.I. = (1.004; 1.034)). Moreover, we noted that the OR of *bad performances*, although decreased in models 2 and 3, in model 4 it assumed the same value of that in model 1, and slightly different in model 4a (overlapping 95% C.I.).

Table 3. Comparison of the OR and corresponding 95% C.I. of *bad performances*, *total mistakes*, and *mistakes in good performances* for the prediction of *new fallers* in the binary logistic regression models.

	New Fallers								
	Bad Performances			Total Mistakes			Mistakes in Good Performances		
	OR	95% C.I.	p	OR	95% C.I.	p	OR	95% C.I.	p
Model 1	1.114	1.040–1.194	0.002	1.014	1.007–1.021	<0.001	1.016	1.007–1.026	<0.001
Model 2	1.090	1.013–1.173	0.021	1.012	1.003–1.022	0.009	1.011	0.998–1.025	0.095
Model 3	1.076	0.998–1.160	0.057	1.008	0.998–1.018	0.123	1.003	0.990–1.017	0.646
Model 4	1.114	1.026–1.211	0.011	1.008	0.998–1.019	0.131	0.999	0.984–1.014	0.914
Model 4a	1.110	1.021–1.207	0.014	1.008	0.997–1.019	0.159	0.999	0.983–1.014	0.855

Models for each main predictor, i.e., *bad performances*, *total mistakes*, or *mistakes in good performances*: model 1, with just the main predictor; model 2, adjusted with mean RT and SD RT; model 3, which was model 2 with the addition of age, sex, and education level; model 4, the fully adjusted regression model, considering also all the other covariates mentioned in Section 2.1.5 (anxiety, depression, hypertensives, diabetes, smoking, alcohol, and IPAQ); and model 4a, which was model 4 adjusted by UGS at baseline (wave 1). The odds ratio (OR) and corresponding 95% confidence interval (C.I.) give a measure of the influence of the predictor on the outcome; the *p*-value expresses the statistical significance of the predictor in the model.

3.4. Comparison with Other Potential Predictors

Table 2 shows a comparison of the OR, reporting also the 95% C.I. and *p*-value, for the three predictors in the five different logistic regression models, as defined in Section 2.3.1. In each model, all predictors were significantly associated with the outcome *TUG decline*. However, the variable *bad performances* always had a larger OR than that of other predictors, and without overlap of 95% C.I.s, suggesting its larger weight in the prediction of this outcome.

Table A6 in Appendix A shows the results for the prediction of the other variable expressing mobility decline, *UGS decline*, in all four binary logistic regression models for each of the three main potential predictors: *bad performances*, *total mistakes* and *mistakes in good performances*. In models 3 and 4, none of the three predictors were significantly associated with the *UGS decline*, while *bad performances* was significant in model 1, and *total mistakes* and *mistakes in good performances* were significant in models 1 and 2. We note that in model 1 *bad performances* had the highest OR with non-overlapping 95% C.I. compared to *total mistakes* and *mistakes in good performances*.

We repeated the procedure for the outcome *new faller*, and the results of the comparison are shown in Table 3. Again, the independent variable *bad performances* performed better than the other two predictors in model 1, having a larger OR and a non-overlapping C.I. In model 3, the *p*-value for *bad performances* was borderline ($|p - 0.05| < 0.01$), while for *total mistakes* and *mistakes in good performances* it was statistically insignificant ($p \gg 0.05$). In models 4 and 4a, *bad performances* emerged as the only variable that was statistically significant for the prediction of *new faller*, with OR = 1.114 in model 4, i.e., for every one-unit increase in *bad performances* we would expect an increase of 0.114 in the odds of becoming a new faller, and OR = 1.110 in model 4a.

Our findings suggested that the independent variable *bad performances* was more predictive of mobility decline and risk of new falls than the other two candidate variables derived from the SART visualisation, i.e., *total mistakes* and *mistakes in good performances*.

3.5. Absence of Association with Cognitive Decline

As shown in Table 4, the variable *bad performances* was not a significant predictor of *MMSE decline* (*p*-value = 0.187) in the fully adjusted model 4, nor in model 4a. *Total mistakes* and *mistakes in good performances* were not significant predictors either in the fully adjusted models. Table A7 in Appendix A shows the results of the binary logistic regression model 4 fully adjusted per covariates considering the independent variable *bad performances* and having as outcome *MMSE decline*. In this case, the only significant predictors were age ($p < 0.001$, OR = 1.044, 95% C.I. = (1.029; 1.059)) and current smoking ($p = 0.013$, OR = 1.523, 95% C.I. = (1.092; 2.123)), both positively associated with increased odds of *MMSE decline*.

Table A8 in Appendix A presents similar results for model 4a, with the only difference that beside age ($p < 0.001$, OR = 1.041, 95% C.I. = (1.025; 1.057)) and current smoking ($p = 0.020$, OR = 1.491, 95% C.I. = (1.066; 2.085)), third or higher education level was significant for the outcome, specifically protective against an *MMSE decline* ($p = 0.043$, OR = 0.738, 95% C.I. = (0.549; 0.991)).

Table 4. Comparison of the OR and corresponding 95% C.I. of *bad performances*, *total mistakes*, and *mistakes in good performances* for the prediction of *MMSE decline* in the binary logistic regression models.

	MMSE Decline								
	Bad Performances			Total Mistakes			Mistakes in Good Performances		
	OR	95% C.I.	p	OR	95% C.I.	p	OR	95% C.I.	p
Model 1	1.120	1.037–1.208	0.004	1.019	1.012–1.027	<0.001	1.026	1.016–1.036	<0.001
Model 2	1.067	0.981–1.159	0.129	1.014	1.004–1.024	0.004	1.019	1.005–1.033	0.006
Model 3	1.030	0.944–1.124	0.503	1.007	0.997–1.017	0.186	1.009	0.995–1.023	0.219
Model 4	1.067	0.969–1.174	0.187	1.010	0.999–1.021	0.082	1.011	0.995–1.026	0.178
Model 4a	1.063	0.965–1.170	0.216	1.010	0.998–1.021	0.090	1.011	0.995–1.027	0.180

Models for each main predictor, i.e., *bad performances*, *total mistakes*, or *mistakes in good performances*: model 1, with just the main predictor; model 2, adjusted with mean RT and SD RT; model 3, which was model 2 with the addition of age, sex, and education level; model 4, the fully adjusted regression model, considering also all the other covariates mentioned in Section 2.1.5 (anxiety, depression, hypertensives, diabetes, smoking, alcohol, and IPAQ); and model 4a, which was model 4 adjusted by UGS at baseline (wave 1). The odds ratio (OR) and corresponding 95% confidence interval (C.I.) give a measure of the influence of the predictor on the outcome; the *p*-value expresses the statistical significance of the predictor in the model.

Table 4 shows the comparison between *bad performances*, *total mistakes*, and *mistakes in good performances* in the prediction of *MMSE decline*, reporting OR, and corresponding 95% C.I and *p*-value for the five binary logistic regression models employed. Of note, all three predictors were significant for *MMSE decline* in model 1 (i.e., where each of the three predictors was the only independent variable in the model), and in this case *bad performances* had the highest OR with non-overlapping 95% C.I. compared to *total mistakes* and *mistakes in good performances*.

4. Discussion

4.1. Multimodal Visualisation

In the present study, we devised a new methodology for the multimodal visualisation of big repeated-measures data with continuous variable ordering and categorical stratification, and we exemplified this with the case of raw SART performance data, accompanied by MMSE and TUG values, sorted by age, and stratified by baseline TUG performance.

By using this novel type of visualisation, clinicians could gain a deeper understanding as to how a complex repeated-measures dataset is articulated across different subjects and across repeated measures (SART trials in this case). Moreover, using the ordering of a continuous variable (age in this case) in the whole dataset (Figure 1) and within each category (Figure 2) allows one to compare the performance of different subjects by age and to formulate hypotheses that can then be tested with formal statistical analyses. Furthermore, by using the threshold for bad performance (Figures 1b and 2b) one can more clearly visualise their distribution across subjects and RTs. This could be the first step in the formulation of a new model to assign cognitive scores to different individuals based on the co-existence of a wide range of different types of parameters.

The visualisations helped us quickly appreciate that bad performances were rare in younger participants (i.e., in their 50s) and concentrated around lower RTs, while in older subjects (i.e., in their 70s and 80s), a wider distribution of bad performances was suggested across a wider range of RTs. By using the thresholding visualisation method, we were able to gain a more focused insight into the participants who had bad SART performances and cross-inspect them with corresponding global parameters of clinical interest such as the total number of SART mistakes, MMSE, and TUG values.

Indeed, the most important characteristic of our visualisation method is the possibility to rapidly visualise raw data and gain immediate insights as to the possible correlations with different kinds of parameters. This multimodal raw data inspection can help visually identify anomalies and outliers in the data, in a way that is diluted and often undetected in traditional designs based on average measures. For example, a high peak in the total mistakes line can be due to one bad performance or multiple performances with just 1 or 2 mistakes, which, in our case would not be labelled as "bad performance" since our threshold required 4 mistakes for the definition of a "bad performance". The superimposed MMSE and TUG curves further underscore multi-modality by providing a global cognitive and mobility score for each participant. The possibility to look at them together with the whole distribution of SART RT values (not just derivative global variables for SART) can provide a more nuanced understanding of the combined cognitive and mobility status of an individual.

Raw data visualisation can therefore support the generation of multiple novel hypotheses involving the relationship between test performance features and other modalities of clinical interest. For example, in our visualisations it was clear that longer TUG times corresponded to higher concentrations of bad performances, and even to the biggest spots among bad performances, i.e., those with very high number of mistakes (biggest light blue spots in Figure 2b). Moreover, we could notice that 'dips' in MMSE seemed to have a very modest association with SART RT performance [51]. Not only were the lowest MMSE scores generally not in correspondence with the high number of total SART mistakes, they were not even present among participants with bad performances, as can be seen comparing panels (a) and (b) in Figure 2. Therefore, we directed our interest towards investigating possible associations between SART bad performances at wave 1 and risk of mobility and/or cognitive decline at wave 3 after 4 years.

4.2. Individual Trial Mistake Threshold in Longitudinal Analysis–Mobility Decline

The cross-sectional considerations on possible associations among SART performance, mobility, and cognitive status, which emerged from the multimodal visualisation, were explored in this study at a longitudinal level. A great advantage of the TILDA study is that it allows for the investigation of variation in certain variables over time, thanks to data being collected longitudinally across different waves [16,21,25].

The longitudinal power of the TILDA study has been used in many recent works aiming to understand correlations between different physiological systems and formulate hypotheses on the possible prediction of mobility and/or cognitive decline [21,24,25]. However, the precise mechanisms governing the longitudinal relationship between cognitive and mobility status are still unclear.

Gait disorders and mobility impairment are very common in older adults [34,52], and are often related to neurological diseases [53,54]. Current literature suggests the presence of correlations between cognitive and motor function in older adults [25,55]; specifically, it has been shown that gait abnormalities could precede and predict the onset of cognitive decline [56,57]. Various standard measures of cognitive status have been used in recent studies, usually in the form of derived variables that while giving a simplified insight on complex repeated-measures data, could carry the risk of losing relevant primary information [5,24]. Recent findings have demonstrated that baseline mobility, expressed by gait parameters and TUG were not significant predictors of cognitive decline in community-dwelling older adults who were cognitively intact at baseline [24]. However, other recent works [22,23] have shown significant associations between baseline quantitative gait parameters and risk of cognitive decline and dementia. Investigating the aforementioned correlations in the opposite direction, recent longitudinal studies [25] suggested that longer motor response time in a choice reaction test could be a significant predictor of accelerated mobility decline, although this effect was statistically and clinically small.

Furthermore, recent studies have shown associations between variability in SART and risk of falls and falls efficacy [17]. Falls are very common amongst older persons [58,59], affecting them not only in the moment of the fall itself, but also later with irreversible consequences, especially in people living with higher levels of frailty [60,61]. Consequences may not only be physical, but also psychological, since some fallers often voluntarily reduce their movements after falling fearing to fall again, and this eventually leads to deconditioning and weakness that in turn increase the risk of further falls [62].

In our study, we aimed to introduce not only a visualisation that would shed light on the whole information contained in a complex dataset like SART, but also individuate a subset of participants containing key information to predict mobility decline and risk of falls in older adults. We considered the outliers for 2 SD from the mean of the distribution of the number of mistakes committed across the different SART trials and across all participants. Such outliers' trials were labelled as "bad performances" if the participant committed at least four mistakes out of nine possible correct actions. The new thresholding method individuated a new variable expressing the number of bad performances for each participant. We noted that only 565 participants had at least 1 bad performance, compared to the whole cohort at wave 1 of 4864 participants. Therefore, the subset defined by the threshold was only the 11.6% of the entire dataset, and we hypothesised that the defined subset could contain valuable information to predict the risk of mobility decline.

We considered the temporal evolution of mobility status, expressed by TUG, UGS, and history of falls at waves 1 and 3, and found that not only the distributions of *TUG/UGS/falls* at the two waves were statistically significantly different from each other, but significant differences were also found for longitudinal TUG increment ($TUG_3 - TUG_1$) and longitudinal UGS decrease ($UGS_1 - UGS_3$) between the subgroup of participants with only good SART performances at wave 1 and participants with at least one SART bad performance. Further investigating this, we found that our new SART variable *bad performances* was a significant predictor of *TUG decline* in the employed binary logistic regression models, being associated with an increase per unit of around 30% in the odds of having TUG decline in the fully adjusted models. Moreover, and consistently with previous literature on cardiovascular burden and mobility limitations in older adults [63], we noted that in model 4, advancing age, the presence of antihypertensives and diabetes, and current smoking status were significant positive predictors of *TUG decline*, bringing an increase in the probability for the outcome of about 14%, 94%, 68%, and 79%, respectively. Moreover, in keeping with the literature [64] and clinical expectation, a significant negative predictor of *TUG decline* was a high level of self-reported physical activity, which decreased by 32% the probability of *TUG decline*. However, considering also UGS at baseline as a covariate in model 4a we noted that some independent variables lost significance in the prediction of *TUG decline*; the only significant positive predictors were *bad performances*, advancing age, and antihypertensive medication use, which determined an increase of 30%, 10%, and 67%, respectively, on the probability of the outcome, while higher UGS at wave 1 was protective against *TUG decline*, leading to a decrease of 6% in the probability. We note that the difference of results between models 4 and 4a were probably due to the high correlation between UGS_1 and TUG_1, and between UGS_3 and TUG_3 (Spearman's correlation coefficient $|\rho| \geq 0.700$ at the significance level of 0.01). Therefore, it was highly probable that UGS at baseline would influence the probability of having a TUG decline after 4 years. Nevertheless, we note that even considering a variable strongly associated with the outcome, *bad performances* did not lose its significance, demonstrating it to be a robust predictor of *TUG decline*.

Our findings suggested that participants with SART bad performances and with a normal TUG at wave 1 ($TUG_1 < 12$ s) had a 30% greater probability to have a TUG at wave 3 indicating a mobility impairment (i.e., $TUG_3 \geq 12$ s). Moreover, comparing the contribution of *bad performances* in the five models employed, we noticed that (i) even adding covariates, it remained a significant predictor, suggesting its robustness in the prediction of the outcome, and (ii) although its OR decreased in models 2 and 3 compared to model 1, it increased again in model 4, and even more in model 4a. The latter observation suggests that in models 2 and 3, other covariates significantly influenced the probability of the outcome, however these variables were not robust for the model, since the presence of further covariates in model 4 and 4a made their presence not significant for the model. In this case, *bad performances* remained significant and regained part of the prediction power temporarily lost in model 3. Furthermore, considering model 4a, where a variable (*UGS*) highly correlated to the outcome was used as a covariate, *bad performances* not only did not lose significance, but also its prediction power increased further, taking part of the weight from less robust independent variables, which were significant predictors in model 4.

Equivalently, we employed the first four logistic regression models for the prediction of *UGS decline*. In this case, *bad performances* was a significant predictor only in model 1, but was not significant in the fully adjusted model. To explain the difference in the results between *TUG decline* and *UGS decline*, we need to understand how these two mobility measures were taken. To measure UGS, participants were required to simply walk in a straight line. This task, then, does not require any major cognitive involvement, since walking is an action that is normally executed automatically in independent adults. Differently, TUG task requires participants to stand up, walk in a straight line, come back, and sit again. Thus, this test is more cognitively involved than straight-line walking, as the individual needs to process and remember instructions, plan and execute movements, focus on the task, and avoid distractions [20]. SART *bad performances* could capture cognitive processes that are similar to those required for completion of the TUG, and this could be a possible explanation as to why *bad performances* independently predicted future mobility decline in our analyses.

Similarly, we considered SART *bad performances* as one of the independent variables in binary logistic regression models for the prediction of becoming a new faller at wave 3. We found that our new variable was a significant positive predictor in the fully adjusted models. In fact, the presence of SART *bad performances* in participants who did not have any falls at wave 1 contributed to an 11% additional probability of falls at wave 3, compared to those who did not have any SART bad performances at wave 1, i.e., who never hit the threshold of 4 mistakes in one trial. We noted that among all the other covariates used in the model, only age was a significant predictor of becoming a new faller at wave 3, although with a low positive contribution of only 2% to the odds of the outcome. Even in this case, comparing the *bad performances* contribution in the five models employed, we observed a phenomenon similar to that for the prediction of *TUG decline*. Indeed, we could notice a decrease in its prediction power in models 2 and 3 with additional loss of significance in model 3 due to the presence of significant predictors among the added covariates. However, in model 4 and 4a it reacquired significance and predictive weight, suggesting the non-robustness of previously significant covariates.

Comparison with Traditional SART Measures as Predictors

Traditional SART variables measure global features, such as the total number of mistakes (omission and/or commission errors) in the whole task, and the mean RT and SD RT across the whole task [5,17,20,24,44]. However, using global parameters, which average a large complex dataset, such as the SART, important information residing in individual trials in the set of repeated measures may be lost. Indeed, no significant associations between SART global parameters and mobility status had been previously found [17,24]; and even when correlations involving reaction time measures had been found, the statistical effect was quite small [25].

In the present study, we aimed to define a new variable, which, being more selective, could discriminate the participants with greater risk of mobility decline. We demonstrated that our variable *bad performances* was a significant predictor of risk of TUG decline and becoming a new faller. Furthermore, we compared its predictive power with other potential predictors: the global parameter *total mistakes* and *mistakes in good performances*, obtained by summing up all the mistakes in SART good performances, i.e., where the maximum number of mistakes per trial was less than 4. We noted that the variables *bad performances* and *mistakes in good performances* were almost complementary, because *mistakes in good performances* considers all the mistakes that are not reaching the threshold for the definition of a bad performance.

In the literature, there is not a uniform consensus on the method to follow in order to compare the importance of different predictors in binary logistic regression [21,65,66]. We compared the models with the different potential predictors for *TUG decline*, *UGS decline*, and *new fallers* considering the OR with non-overlapping 95% C.I. when the independent variable was significant for the prediction of the outcome.

In the fully adjusted models for the prediction of *TUG decline*, we found that, although all three variables considered were significant as predictors, the new variable *bad performances* had a higher OR compared to *total mistakes* and *mistakes in good performances*, where the difference between ORs considering the C.I. was equal or greater than 0.092 in model 4, and 0.083 in model 4a. Specifically, while the effect of the variable *bad performances* per unit was around 30% on the probability of the outcome, *total mistakes*, and *mistakes in good performances* had an effect per unit of only 3% on the probability of the outcome, namely 1 magnitude less than *bad performances*.

Regarding the prediction of *UGS decline*, no SART-related variables were significant as predictors for the outcome in the fully adjusted model. *Bad performances, total mistakes*, and *mistakes in good performances* were all significant in model 1, where *bad performances* assumed the highest OR, and *total mistakes* and *mistakes in good performances* were also significant in model 2, but they all lost their significance in models adjusted for covariates. This result may be due to the fact that, while UGS is a simpler measure of physical mobility, the TUG task is more cognitively involved and, thus, logistic regression models were able to detect the correlation with SART variables.

Moreover, we found that *bad performances* significantly predicted *new falls*, i.e., falls at wave 3 for participants who did not have any falls at wave 1, while *total mistakes* and *mistakes in good performances* were not significant predictors. Namely, our findings suggested that for participants who did not report any falls at wave 1, the number of mistakes in SART task was not a risk of falls at wave 3, as long as they did not hit the threshold of 4 mistakes in a single trial.

Furthermore, comparing the three predictors' performance across the five models employed, we noticed that in the prediction of both *TUG decline* and risk of becoming a new faller, the predictors' *total mistakes* and *mistakes in good performances* did not manifest the same phenomenon observed for *bad performances*. Namely, the presence of covariates in models 2 and 3 was associated with a decrease in prediction power, expressed by the OR, of *total mistakes* and *mistakes in good performances* for both outcomes, with additional loss of significance in model 3 for *total mistakes* and models 2 and 3 for *mistakes in good performances* in the prediction of *new fallers*. Differently from the models involving *bad performances*, in this case in model 4 and 4a the predictors did not reacquire prediction power nor significance for the prediction of *new fallers*, suggesting that they were not robust and strong enough in the prediction, and possibly other covariates revealed to be significant in the model.

Our results suggest that when SART mistakes reach threshold status, the number of times that this happens should be taken seriously as potentially heralding mobility decline and/or falls; however, mistakes below threshold level were less predictive and this could be used to reassure participants that 'one swallow does not make a spring' when it comes to interpreting the clinical significance of a participant making sub-threshold mistakes during the SART task. This still agrees with the principle that clinicians who administer tests of neurocognitive performance (such as the SART) should be reluctant to attribute poor test performance to anxiety that occurs during the testing process [67], but at the same time argues in favour of not placing undue emphasis on the clinical significance of mistakes that occur below a proven threshold. Interestingly, anxiety was not a significant covariate in any of the fully adjusted logistic regression models, which further dilutes the potential mechanistic role of anxiety in the prediction of the four clinical outcomes under study. Another interesting insight from our analyses is that once the focus was on the new visualisation features and additional covariates, mean SART RT and SD of RT had no independent effect on the prediction of any of the outcomes. Since RT variables have been the main focus of previous research on SART-related health outcomes, we would support the need to revisit those studies fort the potential effects of thresholded error features as reported herein.

4.3. Individual Trial Mistake Threshold in Longitudinal Analysis–Cognitive Decline

SART and MMSE are two standard tests used to evaluate cognitive functions: the first specifically measures the sustained attention, the ability to be vigilant over time, and the second gives a more global score on the cognitive status [27]. Cross-sectional studies have suggested only modest associations between SART performance, considering traditional measures, and MMSE score [51,68]. In our study, we investigated the predictive ability of our new variable SART *bad performances* and other independent variables *total mistakes* and *mistakes in good performances* for cognitive decline, expressed by a decline on MMSE score of at least 2 points after 4 years. We found that all three variables considered were not significant predictors of *MMSE decline* in the fully adjusted models. We note that, similarly to previous works [24], a decline in MMSE score was very hard to detect at wave 3 in our sample for different reasons: (i) the participants attending the TILDA health assessment centre (where the SART test was administered) were relatively high-functioning community-dwelling adults with good cognitive and physical health [69]; (ii) the MMSE test performed at each wave has always the same structure, and therefore participants can show learning effects potentially resulting in even higher MMSE scores over time and absence of general decline [70,71]. To overcome this potential limitation, future work could investigate these correlations over a longer time period, or with different global cognitive tests.

4.4. Strengths and Limitations of the Study

One of the main strengths of our study is the large dataset and comprehensive health assessment; indeed, TILDA is one of the most detailed population-based longitudinal studies of ageing, and the comprehensive measures and tests taken at different waves constitute the main strength for longitudinal analyses involving various physiological systems. Specifically, the complex SART dataset offers the possibility of investigating repeated measures for a large sample of individuals. As discussed above, the multimodal visualisation carried out in the present study allows to easily observe the large sample organised by age, stratified by categories of interest, and allow visual associations with other measures included in the health assessment. The new threshold feature based on SART single trials, is not only easy to determine by clinicians, but also offers a meaningful measure to identify subjects at risk of mobility decline over a 4-year period. As done with other types of data [72], this novel visualisation methodology could form the basis of a web-based platform able to facilitate each of the mentioned processes by integrating the different phases into an intuitive system with a graphical user interface that hides the complexity underlying each of the data modalities used, and presents the results in a flexible and visual way, avoiding any manual handling of data during the process.

Our study also has potential limitations, for example in the individuation of outliers in the distribution of single trial mistakes across all participants. Many studies [73,74] prefer to remove outliers present in a distribution, because this is not considered to be a good representation of the sample population. However, our analyses demonstrated that, although the subset of participants individuated by the new threshold was relatively small compared to the entire sample, it could serve for the prediction of mobility decline with a good statistical power, and even better than traditional global parameters usually used to characterize the mistakes in SART performances. Another limitation is that the analytical wave 1 sample was only based in TILDA participants who attended the health assessment centre and, as such, findings cannot be considered as necessarily representative of the entire Irish community-dwelling population. In this regard, given the "healthy participant effect" associated with attendance to the health assessment centre [69], together with the 4-year attrition effect, it is possible that our findings may have somehow underestimated the ability of the new SART features to predict mobility decline, new falls, and even cognitive decline. It would be therefore important to attempt to replicate this study in frailer cohorts in the future.

5. Conclusions

In conclusion, the multimodal visualisation carried out in the present study allowed us (i) to appreciate the richness present in the complex raw SART data, which can be otherwise lost using derivative variables; (ii) to rapidly visually inspect a large amount of data; and (iii) inspect the dataset together with different health variables of clinical interest in order to generate hypotheses. In this representation, we were able to look at the entire dataset and compare the participants' performances (between each other) by age; we were also able to correlate the single performance in each trial with global parameters such as number of total mistakes, MMSE and TUG, aiming to have a comprehensive visual overview of the cognitive and physical status of each subject. Based on the visualisation, a newly defined mistakes threshold for individual SART trials was statistically validated. The determined subset presented higher risk of future mobility decline, as measured by *TUG decline*, and falls with a larger statistical effect than other candidate measures, and could therefore be used to identify early signs of health disorders and prioritise individualised clinical interventions to lower the risks. A threshold approach to the evaluation of SART performance in older adults may better identify subjects at higher risk of future mobility decline and/or falls.

Author Contributions: Conceptualisation, R.R. and R.R.-O.; methodology, R.R. and R.R.-O.; software, R.R.; validation, R.R., S.P.K., J.R.C.D and R.R.-O.; formal analysis, R.R.; investigation, R.R., S.P.K., J.R.C.D., E.D. and R.R.-O.; resources, R.A.K. and R.R.-O.; data curation, R.R. and L.N.; writing—original draft preparation, R.R. and R.R.-O.; writing—review and editing, R.R., S.P.K., J.R.C.D., L.N., E.D., R.A.K. and R.R.-O.; visualisation, R.R.; supervision, R.R.-O.; project administration, R.A.K. and R.R.-O.; funding acquisition, R.A.K. and R.R.-O. All authors have read and agreed to the published version of the manuscript.

Funding: This research was funded by Science Foundation Ireland (SFI), grant number 18/FRL/6188. The Irish Longitudinal Study on Ageing (TILDA) is funded by Atlantic Philanthropies, the Irish Department of Health and Irish Life.

Institutional Review Board Statement: The study was conducted according to the guidelines of the Declaration of Helsinki and approved by the Health Sciences Research Ethics Committee of Trinity College Dublin (Wave 1 protocol reference: "The Irish Longitudinal Study on Ageing", approval granted 2 May 2008; Wave 3 protocol reference: "Main Wave 3 Tilda Study", approval granted 9 June 2014).

Informed Consent Statement: Informed consent was obtained from all subjects involved in the study.

Data Availability Statement: The datasets generated during and/or analysed during the current study are not publicly available due to data protection regulations, but are accessible at TILDA on reasonable request. The procedures to gain access to TILDA data are specified at https://tilda.tcd.ie/data/accessing-data/ (accessed on 14 January 2021).

Acknowledgments: The authors would like to acknowledge the continued commitment and cooperation of the TILDA participants and research team.

Conflicts of Interest: The authors declare no conflict of interest. The funders had no role in the design of the study; in the collection, analyses, or interpretation of data; in the writing of the manuscript; or in the decision to publish the results.

Appendix A
SART RT Representation

An arithmetic average $\overline{RT}^v$ was computed for each trial v, where $v = 1, \ldots, 23$, and considering non-null values only (i.e., excluding null values corresponding to the appearance of digit 3 on the screen). Therefore, we only considered the times when the participant correctly pressed the key, according to

$$\overline{RT}^v = \frac{1}{M_v} \sum_{i=1}^{M_v} RT_i^v, \tag{A1}$$

where $M_v \in \{1, \ldots, 9\}$ is the number of times that the participant correctly pressed the key in the trial v, or correctly did not press the key.

SART performance is known to be influenced by age [44], and therefore we recorded the age of participants and ordered the visualisations by increasing age as a continuous variable.

The $\overline{RT}^v \, \forall v \in \{1, \ldots, 23\}$ are plotted in a cloud plot (Figure 1) where the coordinates of each spot were given by the participant index in the age-sorted ascending order (x-coordinate) and by the $\overline{RT}^v$ for each trial v, having then a total of 23 spots for each participant at the same point on the x-axis. The x-axis did not linearly follow the age variable, but it presented the age-sorted participants sequentially and equally spaced. For ease of interpretation, ticks were created to indicate a 5-year age change. Trials where the participant did not press the key at any time and/or some RT were missing did not have the computed average $\overline{RT}^v$ and were, thus, not plotted in the graph. The size of each spot $s_v \forall v \in \{1, \ldots, 23\}$ for each participant was given by

$$s_v = r_v^{-1}, \; r_v = \frac{M_v}{9}, \tag{A2}$$

where r_v is the ratio of the number of times that the key was correctly pressed (or not pressed) over the maximum possible number of correct pressing actions in the trial v, i.e., 9. Therefore, bigger spots correspond to trials with higher number of mistakes. Moreover, the spots are colour-coded based on their size, i.e., the number of mistakes in the corresponding trial, going from light brown (0 mistakes) to black for the maximum number of mistakes (8 mistakes since in the case of 9 mistakes it is not possible to compute the mean RT and then assign a y-coordinate to the spot). Spots with size larger than 2 SD from the mean size $\bar{s}$ calculated across all the trials and all the participants (excluding missing data and trials with 0 correct actions), namely when the number of correct actions for the trial v for the i-th participant was

$$M_{v,i} = \frac{9}{\bar{s} + 2SD} \tag{A3}$$

were highlighted by white edges in the graph and labelled as "big spots". The size $s_{v,i}$ of each spot was scaled by a factor of 4 for clearer representation in the graph.

Table A1. Results for the fully adjusted per covariates binary logistic regression model 4 considering *bad performances* as potential predictor and having *TUG decline* as outcome.

Independent Variable	TUG Decline		
	OR	95% C.I.	p-Value
Bad performances	1.287	1.137–1.456	<0.001
SART mean RT	1.001	0.999–1.002	0.340
SART SD RT	1.003	1.000–1.006	0.080
Age	1.136	1.115–1.159	<0.001
Females	1.171	0.863–1.590	0.311

Table A1. Cont.

	TUG Decline		
Independent Variable	OR	95% C.I.	p-Value
Education level - primary/none - secondary - third/higher	[ref] 0.930 0.985	 0.646–1.337 0.682–1.423	 0.695 0.936
Anxiety	1.030	0.983–1.081	0.217
Depression	1.014	0.990–1.038	0.249
Antihypertensives	1.942	1.451–2.600	<0.001
Diabetes	1.678	1.051–2.680	0.030
Smoker - never - past - current	[ref] 1.012 1.790	 0.743–1.380 1.147–2.795	 0.938 0.010
Drinking problem - "No" - "Don't know" - "Yes"	[ref] 0.676 0.989	 0.197–2.313 0.626–1.564	 0.532 0.964
IPAQ - low - medium - high	[ref] 0.802 0.684	 0.572–1.125 0.474–0.986	 0.201 0.042

Table A2. Results for the fully adjusted per covariates binary logistic regression model 4a considering *bad performances* as potential predictor and having *TUG decline* as outcome.

	TUG Decline		
Independent Variable	OR	95% C.I.	p-Value
Bad performances	1.305	1.130–1.508	<0.001
SART mean RT	1.000	0.999–1.002	0.791
SART SD RT	1.003	1.000–1.007	0.074
Age	1.102	1.080–1.125	<0.001
Females	0.891	0.646–1.231	0.485
Education level - primary/none - secondary - third/higher	[ref] 1.075 1.246	 0.732–1.579 0.843–1.841	 0.711 0.270
Anxiety	1.023	0.973–1.075	0.382
Depression	1.007	0.982–1.033	0.570
Antihypertensives	1.672	1.230–2.273	0.001
Diabetes	1.348	0.818–2.220	0.241
Smoker - never - past - current	[ref] 0.951 1.581	 0.685–1.319 0.989–2.529	 0.762 0.056
Drinking problem - "No" - "Don't know" - "Yes"	[ref] 0.660 0.907	 0.178–2.443 0.562–1.463	 0.534 0.689

Table A2. Cont.

	TUG Decline		
Independent Variable	**OR**	**95% C.I.**	**p-Value**
UGS at baseline	0.938	0.928–0.948	<0.001
IPAQ - low - medium - high	[ref] 0.959 0.815	 0.671–1.370 0.554–1.199	 0.819 0.299

Table A3. Results for the fully adjusted per covariates binary logistic regression model 4 considering *bad performances* as potential predictor and having *UGS decline* as outcome.

	UGS Decline		
Independent Variable	**OR**	**95% C.I.**	**p-Value**
Bad performances	1.057	0.903–1.237	0.492
SART mean RT	1.001	0.999–1.003	0.301
SART SD RT	1.003	0.998–1.008	0.241
Age	1.093	1.064–1.122	<0.001
Females	1.178	0.752–1.845	0.474
Education level - primary/none - secondary - third/higher	 [ref] 1.088 1.078	 0.633–1.870 0.615–1.890	 0.761 0.792
Anxiety	0.999	0.932–1.072	0.986
Depression	1.032	0.999–1.066	0.061
Antihypertensives	1.767	1.138–2.745	0.011
Diabetes	1.558	0.794–3.057	0.198
Smoker - never - past - current	 [ref] 0.905 1.351	 0.573–1.427 0.694–2.628	 0.666 0.376
Drinking problem - "No" - "Don't know" - "Yes"	 [ref] 1.849 1.093	 0.537–6.371 0.563–2.121	 0.330 0.793
IPAQ - low - medium - high	 [ref] 0.855 0.657	 0.530–1.379 0.382–1.130	 0.520 0.129

Table A4. Results for the fully adjusted per covariates binary logistic regression model 4 considering *bad performances* as potential predictor and having *New faller* as outcome.

	New Fallers		
Independent Variable	**OR**	**95% C.I.**	**p-Value**
Bad performances	1.114	1.026–1.211	0.011
SART mean RT	0.999	0.998–1.001	0.298
SART SD RT	1.001	0.999–1.004	0.319
Age	1.020	1.006–1.034	0.004

Table A4. *Cont.*

	New Fallers		
Independent Variable	**OR**	**95% C.I.**	***p*-Value**
Females	1.237	0.997–1.536	0.053
Education level - primary/none - secondary - third/higher	[ref] 1.033 1.065	 0.779–1.370 0.799–1.420	 0.821 0.667
Anxiety	1.002	0.969–1.036	0.917
Depression	1.014	0.998–1.031	0.092
Antihypertensives	1.184	0.947–1.481	0.139
Diabetes	1.111	0.741–1.668	0.610
Smoker - never - past - current	[ref] 1.200 1.042	 0.579–2.489 0.769–1.412	 0.624 0.792
Drinking problem - "No" - "Don't know" - "Yes"	[ref] 0.971 0.905	 0.755–1.248 0.697–1.176	 0.816 0.457
IPAQ - low - medium - high	[ref] 1.002 1.014	 0.969–1.036 0.998–1.031	 0.917 0.092

Table A5. Results for the fully adjusted per covariates binary logistic regression model 4a considering *bad performances* as potential predictor and having *New faller* as outcome.

	New Fallers		
Independent Variable	**OR**	**95% C.I.**	***p*-Value**
Bad performances	1.110	1.021–1.207	0.014
SART mean RT	0.999	0.998–1.001	0.278
SART SD RT	1.002	0.999–1.004	0.264
Age	1.019	1.004–1.034	0.011
Females	1.232	0.990–1.534	0.061
Education level - primary/none - secondary - third/higher	[ref] 1.020 1.043	 0.768–1.354 0.781–1.393	 0.892 0.775
Anxiety	1.004	0.971–1.038	0.826
Depression	1.014	0.998–1.031	0.089
Antihypertensives	1.174	0.935–1.474	0.166
Diabetes	1.113	0.736–1.682	0.613
Smoker - never - past - current	[ref] 1.148 1.071	 0.920–1.434 0.768–1.493	 0.222 0.688

Table A5. *Cont.*

	New Fallers		
Independent Variable	OR	95% C.I.	*p*-Value
Drinking problem - "No" - "Don't know" - "Yes"	[ref] 1.206 1.033	 0.581–2.501 0.760–1.403	 0.615 0.837
UGS at baseline	0.999	0.994–1.005	0.851
IPAQ - low - medium - high	[ref] 0.960 0.892	 0.745–1.237 0.685–1.163	 0.751 0.399

Table A6. Comparison of the OR and corresponding 95% C.I. of *bad performances, total mistakes* and *mistakes in good performances* for the prediction of *UGS decline* in the binary logistic regression models.

	UGS Decline								
	Bad Performances			Total Mistakes			Mistakes in Good Performances		
	OR	95% C.I.	*p*	OR	95% C.I.	*p*	OR	95% C.I.	*p*
Model 1	1.232	1.102–1.377	<0.001	1.036	1.024–1.047	<0.001	1.049	1.033–1.066	<0.001
Model 2	1.126	0.993–1.277	0.064	1.025	1.010–1.041	0.002	1.036	1.014–1.060	0.001
Model 3	1.058	0.917–1.222	0.438	1.010	0.993–1.028	0.242	1.016	0.992–1.040	0.205
Model 4	1.057	0.903–1.237	0.492	1.013	0.994–1.033	0.180	1.022	0.995–1.049	0.105

Models for each main predictor, i.e., *bad performances, total mistakes*, or *mistakes in good performances*: model 1, with just the predictor; model 2, adjusted with mean RT and SD RT; model 3, which was model 2 with the addition of age, sex, and education level; model 4, the fully adjusted regression model, considering also the other covariates mentioned in Section 2.1.5 (anxiety, depression, hypertensives, diabetes, smoking, alcohol, and IPAQ). The odds ratio (OR) and corresponding 95% confidence interval (C.I.) give a measure of the influence of the predictor on the outcome; the *p*-value expresses the statistical significance of the predictor in the model.

Table A7. Results for the fully adjusted per covariates binary logistic regression model 4 considering *bad performances* as potential predictor and having *MMSE decline* as outcome.

	MMSE Decline		
Independent Variable	OR	95% C.I.	*p*-Value
Bad performances	1.067	0.969–1.174	0.187
SART mean RT	1.000	0.999–1.002	0.495
SART SD RT	1.001	0.999–1.004	0.334
Age	1.044	1.029–1.059	<0.001
Females	0.819	0.651–1.031	0.090
Education level - primary/none - secondary - third/higher	[ref] 0.797 0.747	 0.600–1.058 0.557–1.001	 0.117 0.051
Anxiety	1.012	0.976–1.049	0.512
Depression	1.011	0.993–1.029	0.239
Antihypertensives	1.104	0.870–1.402	0.416
Diabetes	0.759	0.473–1.217	0.252
Smoker - never - past - current	[ref] 1.075 1.523	 0.844–1.368 1.092–2.123	 0.558 0.013

Table A7. Cont.

	MMSE Decline		
Independent Variable	OR	95% C.I.	p-Value
Drinking problem - "No" - "Don't know" - "Yes"	[ref] 0.717 0.925	 0.280–1.832 0.661–1.293	 0.487 0.647
IPAQ - low - medium - high	[ref] 1.143 1.192	 0.863–1.514 0.895–1.588	 0.350 0.230

Table A8. Results for the fully adjusted per covariates binary logistic regression model 4a considering *bad performances* as potential predictor and having *MMSE decline* as outcome.

	MMSE Decline		
Independent Variable	OR	95% C.I.	p-Value
Bad performances	1.063	0.965–1.170	0.216
SART mean RT	1.000	0.999–1.002	0.559
SART SD RT	1.001	0.998–1.004	0.375
Age	1.041	1.025–1.057	<0.001
Females	0.816	0.647–1.029	0.086
Education level - primary/none - secondary - third/higher	[ref] 0.792 0.738	 0.596–1.053 0.549–0.991	 0.108 0.043
Anxiety	1.012	0.976–1.049	0.535
Depression	1.011	0.993–1.029	0.233
Antihypertensives	1.093	0.858–1.392	0.471
Diabetes	0.738	0.455–1.197	0.218
Smoker - never - past - current	[ref] 1.070 1.491	 0.840–1.363 1.066–2.085	 0.584 0.020
Drinking problem - "No" - "Don't know" - "Yes"	[ref] 0.714 0.911	 0.279–1.825 0.650–1.278	 0.482 0.590
UGS at baseline	0.998	0.991–1.004	0.436
IPAQ - low - medium - high	[ref] 1.125 1.203	 0.848–1.494 0.902–1.606	 0.414 0.209

References

1. Gualtieri, C.T. Dementia screening using computerized tests. *J. Insur. Med.* **2004**, *36*, 213–227. [PubMed]
2. Gates, N.J.; Vernooij, R.W.; Di Nisio, M.; Karim, S.; March, E.; Martinez, G.; Rutjes, A.W. Computerised cognitive training for preventing dementia in people with mild cognitive impairment. *Cochrane Database Syst. Rev.* **2019**, *3*, CD012279. [CrossRef] [PubMed]
3. Ahn, W.Y.; Busemeyer, J.R. Challenges and promises for translating computational tools into clinical practice. *Curr. Opin. Behav. Sci.* **2016**, *11*, 1–7. [CrossRef]

4. Bertacchini, F.; Rizzo, R.; Bilotta, E.; Pantano, P.; Luca, A.; Mazzuca, A.; Lopez, A. Mid-sagittal plane detection for advanced physiological measurements in brain scans. *Physiol. Meas* **2019**, *40*, 115009. [CrossRef] [PubMed]
5. O'Halloran, A.M.; Finucane, C.; Savva, G.M.; Robertson, I.H.; Kenny, R.A. Sustained attention and frailty in the older adult population. *J. Gerontol. B Psychol. Sci. Soc. Sci.* **2014**, *69*, 147–156. [CrossRef]
6. Song, M.K.; Lin, F.C.; Ward, S.E.; Fine, J.P. Composite variables: When and how. *Nurs. Res.* **2013**, *62*, 45–49. [CrossRef]
7. Robertson, I.H.; Manly, T.; Andrade, J.; Baddeley, B.T.; Yiend, J. "Oops!": Performance correlates of everyday attentional failures in traumatic brain injured and normal subjects. *Neuropsychologia* **1997**, *35*, 747–758. [CrossRef]
8. Paus, T.; Zatorre, R.J.; Hofle, N.; Caramanos, Z.; Gotman, J.; Petrides, M.; Evans, A.C. Time-related changes in neural systems underlying attention and arousal during the performance of an auditory vigilance task. *J. Cogn. Neurosci.* **1997**, *9*, 392–408. [CrossRef]
9. Helton, W.S.; Kern, R.P.; Walker, D.R. Conscious thought and the sustained attention to response task. *Conscious. Cogn.* **2009**, *18*, 600–607. [CrossRef]
10. Mackworth, N.H. Researches on the measurement of human performance. *Res. Meas. Hum. Perform.* **1950**, *268*, 156. [CrossRef]
11. Fassbender, C.; Murphy, K.; Foxe, J.J.; Wylie, G.R.; Javitt, D.C.; Robertson, I.H.; Garavan, H. A topography of executive functions and their interactions revealed by functional magnetic resonance imaging. *Brain Res. Cogn. Brain Res.* **2004**, *20*, 132–143. [CrossRef] [PubMed]
12. O'Connor, C.; Robertson, I.H.; Levine, B. The prosthetics of vigilant attention: Random cuing cuts processing demands. *Neuropsychology* **2011**, *25*, 535–543. [CrossRef] [PubMed]
13. Coull, J.T. Neural correlates of attention and arousal: Insights from electrophysiology, functional neuroimaging and psychopharmacology. *Prog. Neurobiol.* **1998**, *55*, 343–361. [CrossRef]
14. Sturm, W.; de Simone, A.; Krause, B.J.; Specht, K.; Hesselmann, V.; Radermacher, I.; Herzog, H.; Tellmann, L.; Müller-Gärtner, H.W.; Willmes, K. Functional anatomy of intrinsic alertness: Evidence for a fronto-parietal-thalamic-brainstem network in the right hemisphere. *Neuropsychologia* **1999**, *37*, 797–805. [CrossRef]
15. Helton, W.S. Impulsive responding and the sustained attention to response task. *J. Clin. Exp. Neuropsychol.* **2009**, *31*, 39–47. [CrossRef]
16. O'Halloran, A.M.; Fan, C.W.; Kenny, R.A.; Penard, N.; Galli, A.; Robertson, I.H. Variability in sustained attention and risk of frailty. *J. Am. Geriatr. Soc.* **2011**, *59*, 2390–2392. [CrossRef]
17. O'Halloran, A.M.; Penard, N.; Galli, A.; Fan, C.W.; Robertson, I.H.; Kenny, R.A. Falls and falls efficacy: The role of sustained attention in older adults. *BMC Geriatr.* **2011**, *11*, 85. [CrossRef]
18. Bartsch, R.P.; Liu, K.K.; Bashan, A.; Ivanov, P. Network physiology: How organ systems dynamically interact. *PLoS ONE* **2015**, *10*, e0142143. [CrossRef]
19. Rizzo, R.; Zhang, X.; Wang, J.; Lombardi, F.; Ivanov, P.C. Network physiology of cortico-muscular interactions. *Front. Physiol.* **2020**, *11*, 558070. [CrossRef]
20. Donoghue, O.A.; Horgan, N.F.; Savva, G.M.; Cronin, H.; O'Regan, C.; Kenny, R.A. Association between timed up-and-go and memory, executive function, and processing speed. *J. Am. Geriatr. Soc.* **2012**, *60*, 1681–1686. [CrossRef]
21. Briggs, R.; Kennelly, S.P.; Kenny, R.A. Does baseline depression increase the risk of unexplained and accidental falls in a cohort of community-dwelling older people? Data from The Irish Longitudinal Study on Ageing (TILDA). *Int. J. Geriatr. Psychiatry* **2018**, *33*, e205–e211. [CrossRef] [PubMed]
22. Verghese, J.; Wang, C.; Lipton, R.B.; Holtzer, R.; Xue, X. Quantitative gait dysfunction and risk of cognitive decline and dementia. *J. Neurol. Neurosurg. Amp. Psychiatry* **2007**, *78*, 929–935. [CrossRef] [PubMed]
23. Katsumata, Y.; Todoriki, H.; Yasura, S.; Dodge, H.H. Timed up and go test predicts cognitive decline in healthy adults aged 80 and older in okinawa: Keys to Optimal Cognitive Aging (KOCOA) project. *J. Am. Geriatr. Soc.* **2011**, *59*, 2188–2189. [CrossRef]
24. Donoghue, O.; Feeney, J.; O'Leary, N.; Kenny, R.A. Baseline mobility is not associated with decline in cognitive function in healthy community-dwelling older adults: Findings from The Irish Longitudinal Study on Ageing (TILDA). *Am. J. Geriatr. Psychiatry* **2018**, *26*, 438–448. [CrossRef]
25. Chintapalli, R.; Romero-Ortuno, R. Choice reaction time and subsequent mobility decline: Prospective observational findings from The Irish Longitudinal Study on Ageing (TILDA). *EClinicalMedicine* **2021**, *31*, 100676. [CrossRef]
26. Rydalch, G.; Bell, H.B.; Ruddy, K.L.; Bolton, D.A.E. Stop-signal reaction time correlates with a compensatory balance response. *Gait Posture* **2019**, *71*, 273–278. [CrossRef]
27. Folstein, M.F.; Folstein, S.E.; McHugh, P.R. "Mini-mental state". A practical method for grading the cognitive state of patients for the clinician. *J. Psychiatr. Res.* **1975**, *12*, 189–198. [CrossRef]
28. Kearney, P.M.; Cronin, H.; O'Regan, C.; Kamiya, Y.; Savva, G.M.; Whelan, B.; Kenny, R. Cohort profile: The Irish longitudinal study on ageing. *Int. J. Epidemiol.* **2011**, *40*, 877–884. [CrossRef] [PubMed]
29. Donoghue, O.A.; McGarrigle, C.A.; Foley, M.; Fagan, A.; Meaney, J.; Kenny, R.A. Cohort profile update: The Irish Longitudinal Study on Ageing (TILDA). *Int. J. Epidemiol.* **2018**, *47*, 1398. [CrossRef]
30. Briggs, R.; Carey, D.; Kenny, R.A.; Kennelly, S.P. What is the longitudinal relationship between gait abnormalities and depression in a cohort of community-dwelling older people? Data from the Irish Longitudinal Study on Ageing (TILDA). *Am. J. Geriatr. Psychiatry* **2018**, *26*, 75–86. [CrossRef] [PubMed]

31. Arnold, C.M.; Faulkner, R.A. The history of falls and the association of the timed up and go test to falls and near-falls in older adults with hip osteoarthritis. *BMC Geriatr.* **2007**, *7*, 17. [CrossRef] [PubMed]
32. Beauchet, O.; Fantino, B.; Allali, G.; Muir, S.W.; Montero-Odasso, M.; Annweiler, C. Timed up and go test and risk of falls in older adults: A systematic review. *J.Nutr. Health Aging* **2011**, *15*, 933–938. [CrossRef]
33. Miller, M.E.; Magaziner, J.; Marsh, A.P.; Fielding, R.A.; Gill, T.M.; King, A.C.; Kritchevsky, S.; Manini, T.; McDermott, M.M.; Neiberg, R.; et al. Gait speed and mobility disability: Revisiting meaningful levels in diverse clinical populations. *J. Am. Geriatr. Soc.* **2018**, *66*, 954–961. [CrossRef]
34. Sudarsky, L. Gait disorders in the elderly. *N. Engl. J. Med.* **1990**, *322*, 1441–1446. [PubMed]
35. Kenny, R.A.; Coen, R.F.; Frewen, J.; Donoghue, O.A.; Cronin, H.; Savva, G.M. Normative values of cognitive and physical function in older adults: Findings from The Irish Longitudinal Study on Ageing. *J. Am. Geriatr. Soc.* **2013**, *61*, S279–S290. [CrossRef]
36. James, K.; Schwartz, A.W.; Orkaby, A.R. Mobility assessment in older adults. *N. Engl. J. Med.* **2021**, *385*, e22. [CrossRef]
37. O'Connor, D.M.A.; Laird, E.J.; Carey, D.; O'Halloran, A.M.; Clarke, R.; Kenny, R.A.; Molloy, A.M. Plasma concentrations of vitamin B(12) and folate and global cognitive function in an older population: Cross-sectional findings from The Irish Longitudinal Study on Ageing (TILDA). *Br. J. Nutr.* **2020**, *124*, 602–610. [CrossRef]
38. Moriarty, F.; Savva, G.M.; Grossi, C.M.; Bennett, K.; Fox, C.; Maidment, I.; Loke, Y.K.; Steel, N.; Kenny, R.A.; Richardson, K. Cognitive decline associated with anticholinergics, benzodiazepines and Z-drugs: Findings from The Irish Longitudinal Study on Ageing (TILDA). *Br. J. Clin. Pharmacol.* **2021**, *87*, 2818–2829. [CrossRef]
39. Andrews, J.S.; Desai, U.; Kirson, N.Y.; Zichlin, M.L.; Ball, D.E.; Matthews, B.R. Disease severity and minimal clinically important differences in clinical outcome assessments for Alzheimer's disease clinical trials. *Alzheimer's Dement. Transl. Res. Clin. Interv.* **2019**, *5*, 354–363. [CrossRef] [PubMed]
40. Zigmond, A.S.; Snaith, R.P. The hospital anxiety and depression scale. *Acta Psychiatry Scand.* **1983**, *67*, 361–370. [CrossRef] [PubMed]
41. Weissman, M.M.; Sholomskas, D.; Pottenger, M.; Prusoff, B.A.; Locke, B.Z. Assessing depressive symptoms in five psychiatric populations: A validation study. *Am. J. Epidemiol.* **1977**, *106*, 203–214. [CrossRef]
42. Nahler, G. Anatomical therapeutic chemical classification system (ATC). In *Dictionary of Pharmaceutical Medicine*; Springer: Berlin/Heidelberg, Germany, 2009; p. 8.
43. Forde, C. *Scoring the International Physical Activity Questionnaire (IPAQ)*; University of Dublin: Dublin, Ireland, 2018.
44. Carriere, J.S.; Cheyne, J.A.; Solman, G.J.; Smilek, D. Age trends for failures of sustained attention. *Psychol. Aging* **2010**, *25*, 569–574. [CrossRef]
45. Forrester, J.C.; Ury, H.K. The Signed-Rank (Wilcoxon) test in the rapid analysis of biological data. *Lancet* **1969**, *1*, 239–241. [CrossRef]
46. Aizawa, C.Y.P.; Morales, M.P.; Lundberg, C.; Moura, M.C.D.S.D.; Pinto, F.C.G.; Voos, M.C.; Hasue, R.H. Conventional physical therapy and physical therapy based on reflex stimulation showed similar results in children with myelomeningocele. *Arq. Neuro-Psiquiatr.* **2017**, *75*, 160–166. [CrossRef]
47. Domino, E.F.; Caldwell, D.F.; Henke, J.; Henke, R. The differential effects of plasma from two groups of clinically similar schizophrenic patients on learning behavior in rats. *J. Psychiatr. Res.* **1966**, *4*, 87–94. [CrossRef]
48. Le Cessie, S.; Goeman, J.J.; Dekkers, O.M. Who is afraid of non-normal data? Choosing between parametric and non-parametric tests. *Eur. J. Endocrinol.* **2020**, *182*, E1–E3. [CrossRef]
49. Oleckno, W.A.; Anderson, B. *Essential Epidemiology: Principles and Applications*; Waveland Prospect Heights: Prospect Heights, IL, USA, 2002.
50. Greenfield, B.; Henry, M.; Weiss, M.; Tse, S.M.; Guile, J.M.; Dougherty, G.; Zhang, X.; Fombonne, E.; Lis, E.; Lapalme-Remis, S.; et al. Previously suicidal adolescents: Predictors of six-month outcome. *J. Can. Acad. Child. Adolesc. Psychiatry* **2008**, *17*, 197–201. [PubMed]
51. Huntley, J.D.; Hampshire, A.; Bor, D.; Owen, A.M.; Howard, R.J. The importance of sustained attention in early Alzheimer's disease. *Int. J. Geriatr. Psychiatry* **2017**, *32*, 860–867. [CrossRef]
52. Dawson, D.; Hendershot, G.; Fulton, J.; Unwerslty, B. Aging in the eighties. *Funct. Limit. Individ. Age* **1987**, *65*, 1–11.
53. Bloem, B.R.; Haan, J.; Lagaay, A.M.; van Beek, W.; Wintzen, A.R.; Roos, R.A. Investigation of gait in elderly subjects over 88 years of age. *Top. Geriatr.* **1992**, *5*, 78–84. [CrossRef] [PubMed]
54. Fuh, J.-L.; Lin, K.-N.; Wang, S.-J.; Ju, T.-H.; Chang, R.; Liu, H.-C. Neurologic diseases presenting with gait impairment in the elderly. *J. Geriatr. Psychiatry Neurol.* **1994**, *7*, 89–92. [CrossRef] [PubMed]
55. Demnitz, N.; Esser, P.; Dawes, H.; Valkanova, V.; Johansen-Berg, H.; Ebmeier, K.P.; Sexton, C. A systematic review and meta-analysis of cross-sectional studies examining the relationship between mobility and cognition in healthy older adults. *Gait Posture* **2016**, *50*, 164–174. [CrossRef]
56. Verghese, J.; Lipton, R.B.; Hall, C.B.; Kuslansky, G.; Katz, M.J.; Buschke, H. Abnormality of gait as a predictor of non-Alzheimer's dementia. *N. Engl. J. Med.* **2002**, *347*, 1761–1768. [CrossRef] [PubMed]
57. Van Uem, J.M.T.; Walgaard, S.; Ainsworth, E.; Hasmann, S.E.; Heger, T.; Nussbaum, S.; Hobert, M.A.; Micó-Amigo, E.M.; Van Lummel, R.C.; Berg, D.; et al. Quantitative timed-up-and-go parameters in relation to cognitive parameters and health-related quality of life in mild-to-moderate Parkinson's disease. *PLoS ONE* **2016**, *11*, e0151997. [CrossRef]

58. Tinetti, M.E.; Speechley, M.; Ginter, S.F. Risk factors for falls among elderly persons living in the community. *N. Engl. J. Med.* **1988**, *319*, 1701–1707. [CrossRef] [PubMed]
59. Nevitt, M.C.; Cummings, S.R.; Kidd, S.; Black, D. Risk factors for recurrent nonsyncopal falls. A prospective study. *JAMA* **1989**, *261*, 2663–2668. [CrossRef]
60. Greenspan, S.L.; Myers, E.R.; Kiel, D.P.; Parker, R.A.; Hayes, W.C.; Resnick, N.M. Fall direction, bone mineral density, and function: Risk factors for hip fracture in frail nursing home elderly. *Am. J. Med.* **1998**, *104*, 539–545. [CrossRef]
61. Sambrook, P.N.; Cameron, I.D.; Chen, J.S.; Cumming, R.G.; Lord, S.R.; March, L.M.; Schwarz, J.; Seibel, M.J.; Simpson, J.M. Influence of fall related factors and bone strength on fracture risk in the frail elderly. *Osteoporos. Int.* **2007**, *18*, 603–610. [CrossRef]
62. Tinetti, M.E. Preventing falls in elderly persons. *N. Engl. J. Med.* **2003**, *348*, 42–49. [CrossRef]
63. Welmer, A.-K.; Angleman, S.; Rydwik, E.; Fratiglioni, L.; Qiu, C. Association of cardiovascular burden with mobility limitation among elderly people: A population-based study. *PLoS ONE* **2013**, *8*, e65815. [CrossRef]
64. Ferrucci, L.; Cooper, R.; Shardell, M.; Simonsick, E.M.; Schrack, J.A.; Kuh, D. Age-related change in mobility: Perspectives from life course epidemiology and geroscience. *J. Gerontol. Ser. A Biol. Sci. Med Sci.* **2016**, *71*, 1184–1194. [CrossRef]
65. Thomas, D.R.; Zhu, P.; Zumbo, B.D.; Dutta, S. On measuring the relative importance of explanatory variables in a logistic regression. *J. Mod. Appl. Stat. Methods* **2008**, *7*, 4. [CrossRef]
66. Thompson, D. Ranking Predictors in Logistic Regression. Paper D10-2009, 2009. Available online: http://www.mwsug.org/proceedings/2009/stats/MWSUG-2009-D10.pdf (accessed on 25 June 2015).
67. Gass, C.S.; Curiel, R.E. Test anxiety in relation to measures of cognitive and intellectual functioning. *Arch. Clin. Neuropsychol.* **2011**, *26*, 396–404. [CrossRef]
68. Cassarino, M.; Tuohy, I.C.; Setti, A. Sometimes nature doesn't work: Absence of attention restoration in older adults exposed to environmental scenes. *Exp. Aging Res.* **2019**, *45*, 372–385. [CrossRef]
69. Kearney, P.M.; Cronin, H.; O'Regan, C.; Kamiya, Y.; Whelan, B.J.; Kenny, R.A. Comparison of centre and home-based health assessments: Early experience from the Irish Longitudinal Study on Ageing (TILDA). *Age Ageing* **2011**, *40*, 85–90. [CrossRef]
70. Tombaugh, T. Test-retest reliable coefficients and 5-year change scores for the MMSE and 3MS. *Arch. Clin. Neuropsychol.* **2005**, *20*, 485–503. [CrossRef] [PubMed]
71. Feeney, J.; O'Leary, N.; Kenny, R.A. Impaired orthostatic blood pressure recovery and cognitive performance at two-year follow up in older adults: The Irish Longitudinal Study on Ageing. *Clin. Auton. Res.* **2016**, *26*, 127–133. [CrossRef] [PubMed]
72. Benitez, J.A.; Labra, J.E.; Quiroga, E.; Martin, V.; Garcia, I.; Marques-Sanchez, P.; Benavides, C. A web-based tool for automatic data collection, curation, and visualization of complex healthcare survey studies including social network analysis. *Comput. Math. Methods Med.* **2017**, *2017*, 2579848. [CrossRef]
73. Elmougy, S.; Hossain, M.S.; Tolba, A.S.; Alhamid, M.F.; Muhammad, G. A parameter based growing ensemble of self-organizing maps for outlier detection in healthcare. *Clust. Comput.* **2019**, *22*, 2437–2460. [CrossRef]
74. Leidhin, C.N.; McMorrow, J.; Carey, D.; Newman, L.; Williamson, W.; Fagan, A.J.; Chappell, M.A.; Kenny, R.A.; Meaney, J.F.; Knight, S.P. Age-related normative changes in cerebral perfusion: Data from The Irish Longitudinal Study on Ageing (TILDA). *NeuroImage* **2021**, *229*, 117741. [CrossRef]

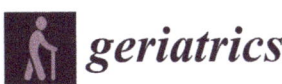

Article

"It Makes You Feel That You Are There": Exploring the Acceptability of Virtual Reality Nature Environments for People with Memory Loss

Noreen Orr [1], Nicola L. Yeo [1], Sarah G. Dean [2], Mathew P. White [3] and Ruth Garside [1,*]

1. European Centre for Environment and Human Health, University of Exeter Medical School, Knowledge Spa, Royal Cornwall Hospital, Truro, Cornwall TR1 3HD, UK; N.Orr@exeter.ac.uk (N.O.); nlyeo@outlook.com (N.L.Y.)
2. Clinical Trials Unit, College of Medicine and Health, University of Exeter, Exeter EX1 1TE, UK; S.Dean@exeter.ac.uk
3. Cognitive Science Hub, University of Vienna, 1110 Vienna, Austria; mathew.white@univie.ac.at
* Correspondence: r.garside@exeter.ac.uk; Tel.: +44-1872-258148

Abstract: Aim: To report on the acceptability of virtual reality (VR) nature environments for people with memory loss at memory cafes, and explore the experiences and perceptions of carers and staff. **Methods:** A qualitative study was conducted between January and March 2019. Ten adults with memory loss, eight carers and six volunteer staff were recruited from two memory cafes, located in Cornwall, UK. There were 19 VR sessions which were audio recorded and all participants were interviewed at the end of the sessions. Framework analysis was used to identify patterns and themes in the data. **Results:** During the VR experience, participants were engaged to varying degrees, with engagement facilitated by the researcher, and in some cases, with the help of a carer. Participants responded positively to the nature scenes, finding them soothing and evoking memories. The VR experience was positive; many felt immersed in nature and saw it as an opportunity to 'go somewhere'. However, it was not always positive and for a few, it could be 'strange'. Participants reflected on their experience of the VR equipment, and volunteer staff and carers also shared their perceptions of VR for people with dementia in long-term care settings. **Conclusions:** The VR nature experience was an opportunity for people with memory loss to be immersed in nature and offered the potential to enhance their quality of life. Future work should build on lessons learned and continue to work with people with dementia in developing and implementing VR technology in long-term care settings.

Keywords: memory loss; virtual reality; technology; nature environments; qualitative research; dementia; long-term care

1. Introduction

Interaction with natural environments, especially marine and coastal, can benefit health and wellbeing [1]. However, many older adults, including those in long-term care, encounter barriers to accessing nature [2] which may contribute to widespread feelings of boredom and depression [3]. How residents might connect with nature to reduce these negative symptoms and improve wellbeing is receiving increased attention from researchers [4]. One possibility is to simulate aspects of nature indoors, enabling access for those residents who may only experience the outdoors infrequently or not at all [5]. Exposure to nature via large TV screens has produced some therapeutic benefits for residents with dementia including improvements in mood [6] and heart rate, a physiological indicator of stress [7]. While more recent work has found that fully immersive head-mounted Virtual Reality (VR) offers even greater benefits than TV [8], there has been a lack of research using totally immersive VR involving older adults with dementia in real world settings [9].

VR can be thought of " ... as a way to relocate people to virtual places and take part in events and activity there" (p. 29, [10]). Participation is key to differentiating VR from other forms of human-computer interaction, in that the person " ... *participates in the virtual world rather than uses it*" (p. 5, [10]). As Heim (p. 70, [11]) puts it, " ... VR *insists* that we move about and physically interact with artificial worlds" (italics added). A special feature of VR is sensory immersion [11] which is the 'technical goal' of VR: to substitute 'real' sensory stimuli (e.g., visual, auditory, olfactory, haptic) with computer-generated ones (p. 4, [10]). However, VR may not achieve this in practice as typically, VR has been primarily an 'optical technology' (p. 1, [12]) with sound sometimes considered. Arguably, visual stimuli are the easiest type of sensory stimuli to replicate in VR and may be sufficient in inducing a sense of immersion by itself in some applications (p. 4, [10,12]), possibly because vision is often regarded as the dominant sense [13]. A combination of technologies such as head-mounted displays, headphones with sound/music, and hand-held controllers providing haptic feedback are used to deliver the immersive VR experience. Ultimately, the aim of a VR experience is 'presence', that feeling of 'being there' in the virtual environment, despite knowing that one is not actually there [14].

There are two primary types of VR: the first is the 360° video made of real scenes filmed with a series of special panoramic lenses facing in different directions that are then brought together to produce a 360° full surround experience; and the second is computer generated images (CGI), often created using gaming engine software. The 360° video represents a relatively passive form of VR with the user observing pre-recorded footage, and requiring little interaction. While greater interaction and immersion is possible with CGI, it is also computationally more demanding and (at least when the study was conducted) requires an accompanying laptop and a heavier, more cumbersome headset. In contrast, the 360° videos can be played on a standard mobile phone placed into a much simpler, lighter and less complicated headset. It was the latter type of VR that was selected for the VR nature experience intervention.

The long-term goal of this research was to develop a VR nature environment intervention for people with dementia living in long-term care facilities. At the study's inception, we were not aware of any research with this population that had specifically trialled exposure to nature by immersive 360-degree videos shown via a head-mounted display. Since the use of VR in healthcare is a relatively recent development, its use with people with dementia is not well understood [9]. There are potentially a number of issues that could limit its use such as cybersickness, fear of, or unwillingness to use, new technology, and the ability to participate and experience presence. Therefore, in order to understand acceptability of VR technology with people with dementia, user testing is crucial (p. 1720, [15]). Before undertaking an extensive formal trial in long-term care settings, we piloted the VR nature experience with older people with mild to moderate memory impairment living in the community. Given that most existing studies on technology and people with dementia acknowledge that the technology is often used as a 'joint activity' in the 'presence of another person' (family member, carer or therapist) [16], we included carers and memory café volunteer staff in our study. In this first attempt to deliver the intervention, acceptability, defined as " ... a subjective evaluation made by individuals who experience ... an intervention" (p. 10, [17]), was assessed during and after delivery.

The aim of the study was to explore the acceptability of VR nature environments for people with memory loss at memory cafes, and explore the experiences and perceptions of carers and volunteer staff. The key research questions for this study were:

- How did older people with mild to moderate cognitive or memory impairment experience the VR nature environments intervention?
- What did carers and volunteer staff facilitating the memory café sessions think about VR for people with dementia and care home residents?

2. Materials and Methods

2.1. Study Design and Participants

Older adults with mild to moderate cognitive or memory impairment, their carers, and volunteer staff were recruited from two memory cafes in Cornwall, South West England. The memory cafes were chosen as a setting for the study because people that attend have memory issues and may or may not have a formal diagnosis of dementia. The researcher (NY) made four visits to each memory café, participated in sessions, and met with the memory café visitors and volunteers to explain the research project to potential participants. All participants provided informed written consent (and the University of Exeter Medical School Ethics Committee reviewed and approved the study (Jan19/B/192)).

2.2. Virtual Reality Nature Intervention

The 360° video VR nature intervention was designed to capture "restorative" nature elements such as gently breaking waves, dappled sunlight on water, thought to innately instil 'soft fascination', hold the viewer's attention effortlessly, and thereby reduce negative emotions, promote relaxation and positive mood states [18]. However, pilot trials revealed that with a lack of 'activity' (e.g., people, animals, movement) in the 360° scenes, users quickly became confused and disengaged as to the purpose of the VR, as they expected 'something to happen'. Given that one of the most problematic issues in long-term care is persistent lack of engagement among residents [19], any intervention should not risk causing further disengagement or confusion. In consultation with memory café chairpersons, we carefully chose clips containing identifiable landmarks, groups of people and interesting, non-threatening wildlife, against a backdrop of 'tranquil' scenery.

The 360° video was a series of 5 × 30 second clips fading into one another, designed to feel like a day's journey through a recognisable local spot, starting in the morning and ending with a sunset. The videos showed pre-recorded scenes of local Cornish beaches and coastal areas with audio of natural sounds such as gently breaking waves. In addition, one video depicted people engaged in activities on a beach with sounds of laughter and chatter. Another clip was taken underwater on a reef that was not local but was of high quality and included footage of gently shoaling fish. Example stills from the clips are shown in Figure 1. There was 'surround sound' rather than headphones to enable the carer to hear and converse with the person with memory loss where needed.

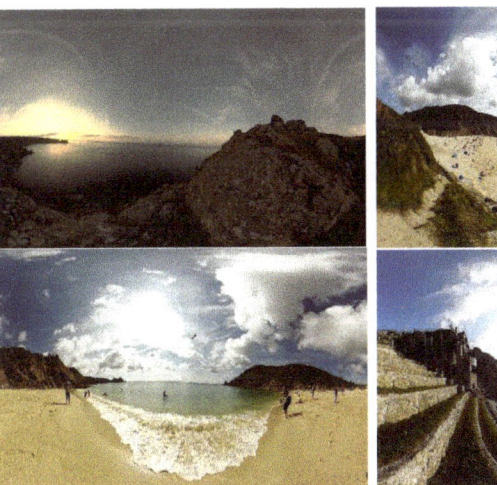
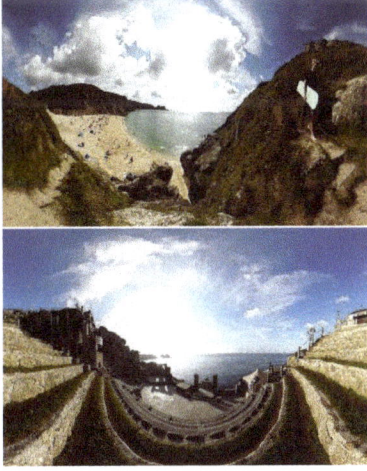

Figure 1. *Cont.*

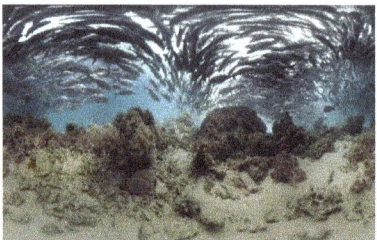

Figure 1. Example stills from each of the 30-second 360° video clips.

The 360° video was played on ZTE Axon 7 smartphone, placed inside a Google Daydream™ VR headset to allow fully panoramic viewing. The smartphone screen had a resolution of 1440 × 2560 pixels (Quad High Definition (QHD)). The smartphone was linked through a wireless connection to a Vodafone N8 Smart Tab 4G tablet using the Showtime VR app, from which the researcher could control the 360° video remotely. This allowed for a more seamless transmission, in which the researcher and carer (where present) could follow the 360° video content on the tablet screen in 'real time', enabling a shared experience. The Daydream headset (Figure 2) was fitted with wipe-clean face cushions which were cleaned with alcohol wipes between individual sessions, and laundered between café visits.

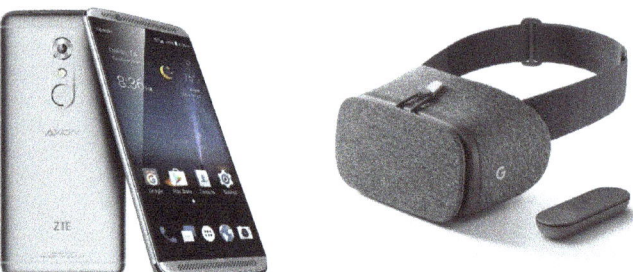

Figure 2. Daydream Headset and ZTE AXON 7 Smartphone.

2.3. Data Collection and Analysis

The video sessions were audio recorded in order to capture 'in the moment' reactions of the participants, sometimes difficult to reproduce in interviews. At the end of the sessions, semi-structured interviews (~10 minutes) were undertaken with the participants to explore perceptions of the of the VR nature experience, experiences of nature and technology, and how VR nature experiences might be suitable for people living with dementia and in long term care. Where both members of the dyad were interviewed together, the initial questions were directed to the person with memory loss, and then subsequently to the carer.

The interviews were recorded and transcribed verbatim. The interview data were analysed using framework analysis [20], commonly used for the thematic analysis of semi-structured interview transcripts. It offers a flexible and systematic approach to analysing qualitative data [21]. Here, it enabled us to combine both deductive and inductive approaches to analysis, with some themes pre-selected based on the literature and the research questions, but open to the possibility of uncovering 'unexpected' themes from the data.

The transcripts were read and re-read, along with the interviewer's reflective notes, as the first step in becoming familiar with the data. This helped to both identify recurring themes and concepts, and devise a conceptual framework of 'main themes'. The next stage involved coding the transcripts and grouping the codes so that data with similar content were brought together. Then, a set of thematic matrices or charts were created which summarised and synthesised the data (Supplementary Tables S1–S5). It remained possible to add additional themes, if required, iteratively throughout the analysis process. Quotes from the participants provide 'thick description' allowing verification of these themes. The findings described below are supported with exemplar quotes and coded as volunteer (V), carer (C), or person with memory loss (ML), along with a numerical code, reflecting their participant number.

3. Results

There were 19 VR sessions at the two memory cafes: four sessions with people with memory loss; three with carers only; six with dyads (comprising an individual living with memory loss and their carer); and six with memory café volunteers (Table 1). Each participant tried the VR experience once.

Table 1. Profile of Participants.

	People with Memory Loss (ML; $n = 10$)	Carers (C; $n = 8$)	Volunteer Staff (V; $n = 6$)
Gender			
Women	6	7	5
Men	4	1	1
Relationship to person with memory loss			
Spouse		5	
Daughter		2	
Friend		1	

Engagement during VR Experience

The participants engaged with the VR nature environments to varying degrees, with many responding with quite detailed descriptions and commentaries on what they were seeing, and others commenting less and attempting to remove the headset before the end of the session. For example, one man with memory loss was animated throughout the experience:

I'm on the beach. Haven't been on the beach in ages! Ooh, it's lovely. Which beach is it, maid*? ... Oh now I'm under the sea! Look at all these fishes. It's good innit? Wow! ... and now there's someone comin' in on a boat. Hello! Ahhh. The waves are lovely (10-ML) [*a Cornish dialect word for girl].

Another participant was similarly engaged and then after one and a half minutes stated that she had had enough:

It's sort of a forest thing, and it's got a path ... like mountains an' that as well. It's very nice ... Oh wow I can see a beach now. Oh yeah, it's a bit like Polzeath it is, with people on it. Oh yeah, people playing games an' that on the beach. It's hot 'cause they got their shorts and t-shirts on. It's very nice. Oh I can see a pink bucket as well. A ... a very busy beach ... very busy ... oh yeah, very nice. [inaudible] they're going out in the boat now. Oh yeah, there's a chap going out on the beach—on the boat now. Ooh, very nice. I've had enough now (05-ML).

There were two others who had limited engagement as they removed the headset a number of times (for example, 07-ML removed the headset after approximately 40 seconds, and 08-ML removed the headset several times during the experience). Engagement was facilitated by the researcher (NY) and in some cases, with the help of a carer. Some carers chose to view the VR nature environments, or part of it, in advance of their partners, to encourage the person with memory loss to participate:

Oh that's under the sea, oh that's looking, oh that's beautiful! Absolutely! Oh we like these sort of things. [husband's name], you'll enjoy this one. The coral, yeah, it's lovely [husband's name]. You'll enjoy that (16-C).

She then continued to encourage her husband to describe what he was seeing and persuaded him to keep the headset on.

Reflections after the VR experience

Participants reflected on their experiences in the interviews after the VR nature experience and six themes are expanded on below, with additional comments from volunteer staff and carers tabulated in Table 2.

Table 2. Volunteer staff and carers' perceptions of VR for Person with Dementia in long-term care.

Perceptions of VR	Illustrative Quote from Volunteer (V) or Carer (C)
1. Alternative means of accessing nature and the outdoors [+]	"I think it's a great idea, especially, like you say, for people who can't get out." (17-C)
	"I think maybe for the person that's being cared for, then yeah. Sort of make them feel like they've got out of the four walls ... even if it's ten minutes." (07-C)
	"sometime in the future, I'll not be able to drive, and I think, if I couldn't get out, that would be great, that sort of thing ... 'Cause it brings the outside back right into you, yeah." (09-V)
2. Relieving boredom [+]	"It gives them a chance to go and see something ... she gets quite bored, and so I think going out to look at something like that, would be quite nice. Whether she'd sit there for long with it on ... but you don't have to do you" (17-C)
3. Trigger memories [+]	"Oh, I think that could be marvellous. If you can make it personal, ... trigger the memories, you know, it would be lovely." (10-C)
	"I think it depends on what sort of dementia they've got, really ... I think it'd be lovely for a lot of people. Especially, as you say, the ones that are in homes. You know, especially if it was a horrible afternoon and you could say 'alright we'll go down to the beach, this is what it was like'. And bringing back memories." (18-V)
	"... if they're able to watch it, I think it'd be brilliant for them. Just like, the way I say, to be able to bring back memories for them. Especially if it was all, sort of, local to that person's ... well, you know, we live in Cornwall, so they're places in Cornwall that we would recognise." (14-V)
4. Improve mood and calming [+]	"I suppose it could help put people in a better mood, especially if they're havin' a bad day, and they can't get out." (10-C)
	"I do think that if someone's having a really bad day, that it would help to calm them. It's like music, 'cause seeing that visually—the sun and people having fun on the beach ... " (06-V)
5. Potentially confusing [−]	"I don't think it would help him [husband LwD]. He'd go through it. He wouldn't remember what had happened two minutes afterwards. I think he might be a bit confused." (02-C)
	"I mean for some people they would find it a bit confusing, you know, and think: 'what on earth's going on here ... this is a bit weird'. Um and especially those who, you know, their memory loss is so great that they don't remember one minute to the next minute ... that contradict themselves all the time you know, so you ask them if they enjoy it one minute and they'd go 'yes', and then you ask them again and they'd go 'what?' ... they can't even remember what they look ... saw" (04-V)

Table 2. *Cont.*

Perceptions of VR	Illustrative Quote from Volunteer (V) or Carer (C)
6. Unable to cope with the VR equipment [−]	"I think one thing about the technology is definitely that [husband] wouldn't be able to cope with it. He would definitely need somebody there to switch it on, switch it off, do whatever is necessary." (03-C)
	"... it's quite heavy on your face, and I think ... it's all going to vary depending on what sort of dementia it is, but I wonder how they would cope moving around, physically and that sort of thing, to see, or whether they would just sort of think they've just gotta look forward. And even, even if they realise they can move around, would they physically be able to do it easily, I don't know?" (14-V)
7. Time-consuming for use in long term care [−]	"I think the sad thing is though ... whether it would actually get used ... in a care setting, I don't know. Because it's time, it's gonna be time consuming isn't it, and it's one-to-one, and everything, and maybe in care settings that's quite a difficult task isn't it, time-wise." (14-V)

[+] Positive; [−] Negative.

3.1. "It Makes You Feel That You Are There": VR as an Immersive Experience

The VR experience often centred around immersion (and presence), and the opportunity to interact with others in a virtual world.

Participants reported that they felt immersed in nature: 'at the sea', 'on the sand' and 'feeling the sand' ("... It looks real, and you feel part of it" [06-V], "... with that, virtually, you're in it, aren't you? It's fantastic" [11-V]):

> Oh, now *I'm in the sea* with the fish! ... Back on the beach. Who's that over there? (13-ML)

> It makes you feel as if you're at the sea, right at the sea, doesn't it? ... it makes you feel that you *are there* [emphasis] on the sand, with the sea rolling in (15-V).

Another volunteer participant reflected on how the VR experience meant 'you were there, in nature':

> and I've got a beautiful view where I live, so I can look out, but I'm looking through a window whereas that [the VR], you're there, which is the difference, yeah (18-V).

One of the participants drew out that the feeling of presence made her 'feel better' as she had difficulty accessing beaches in her everyday life because of reduced mobility:

> Some of these beaches I can't access. So it's actually quite nice to ... see. This actually makes you, it does actually make you feel better 'cause you can sort of, like *it feels like you can feel the sand* [laughs] (19-ML).

Another participant stated:

> I mean it makes you feel, good in a way, you know, just as you can see it, and um, *you don't see anything else*, just all those fishes, the massive fish. (17-ML)

One participant observed that, despite the noisy environment of the memory cafe, she felt that she had 'left' the room, "... closing me ears off to that [the noise]. Concentrating on the panoramic views" (09-V).

A few of the participants found themselves responding to the situations they saw and described how they could have interacted with the people on the beach:

I liked seeing the people on the beach and I liked to, playing the Frisbee thing, you know the one on the beach and he was standing there and I thought, 'well is he gonna talk to me?!' you know [laughs] and I saw the chap in the water catching it and it was just nice to be 'in' there, especially when the surfer came down by your side and went down, it was just like being there (18-V).

3.2. "Oh Beautiful, It Was Lovely": The Soothing Effect of Nature Scenes

All of the participants responded positively to the VR nature experience, typically describing it as 'beautiful' and 'lovely'. It was clear that participants enjoyed nature and appreciated nature 'views' and 'scenery'. Some added that they particularly enjoyed the colours in the scenes ("I've enjoyed looking at them. They're lovely pictures and that. All the colours are beautiful" [01-C], "Oh, very pretty. I love the colours I do. Awww" [05-ML]).

A number of the participants highlighted aspects of the nature scenes that had particular appeal such as the sea, the beach, and the fishes:

The beach and the water coming in and the fish, was lovely [laughs] (08-ML).

Oh that sea, yeah. This is why we came back to Cornwall I think. Well it was, definitely. Incredible sand, isn't it (02-C).

Oh the fishes were beautiful they were. I never been er ... what d'ya call it? ... Diving, I've never done it. But I love the water (10-ML).

Some described these different aspects relaxing and calming:

the sea, the one in the sea was beautiful. Well I like water, for a start. It was just, um, the colours were very beautiful and erm, soothing and um ... I like watching fish (12-ML).

3.3. "It Was Really Nice, Nice to See Places I Recognised": Using Nature to Reminisce

Many of the participants appreciated the familiarity of the scenes and recognised local places in Cornwall:

it was really nice, nice to see places I recognised. I mean it's always nice, when you can identify things—you do it don't you, even when you're watching the telly and that sort of stuff (14-V).

The scenes also prompted many to talk about their past experiences of nature or past experiences in general. One participant said " ... in a way it brings back things to you. You know, going to the seaside, the sea coming in. I think perhaps, that's it, it brings back the memory of it" (06-V), and another stated:

Oh on the beach, you know, because I love the coast, I do. I grew up here in C ... well not here, bit further down, place called Crantock, near Newquay ... spent many a summer holiday in Crantock. My Mother was still there, see. And we took the kids, and then the grandkids when they come along ... It's [the coast] part of me, you know, growin' up with it. I do miss it terribly (13-ML).

Memories could also be tinged with sadness in that the participants realised that there were places that they could no longer enjoy, illustrated by this excerpt from an exchange between a person with dementia and his carer:

16-ML: I took her a lot of places, didn't I maid*? [*a Cornish dialect word for girl]

16-C: Yeah, but I mean, it was interesting to see the different places, an' that

16-ML: Yeah

16-C: Which we won't be seein' anymore, anyhow will we?

One participant with dementia was prompted by the scenes of the underwater coral reefs to recall when he had seen the corals in Egypt in the 1950s. He described how he had been in the British Army doing his National Service and had gone down the Gulf of Suez and swam in the sea where there were "lots of little fishes" and coral (16-ML).

3.4. "It's ... Like Goin on Holiday": VR as a Different Experience

For some participants, the VR experience offered new or different experiences and an opportunity to 'go somewhere':

> but it was lovely 'cause it gives you, I don't know, a sense of freedom, yes. Anyone who's had to be indoors, they just get that feeling of being there. And certainly when it was just the sea, the empty sea, I'd just like to go and have a nice swim (18-V).

> the going under the sea. And just being able to look around like you're walking somewhere—like you're *going* somewhere. It looks, it's really good, yeah (19-ML).

Similarly, seeing the fish evoked a sense of wonder at life underwater ("Oh now I got some fish. Beautiful isn't it? There's so many wonders underneath aren't there, that we don't know about ... hidden treasures" [06-V]), and reminded one participant of the nature documentaries that she and her partner enjoyed:

> we like that coral one. Where you're under the sea. Because we watch those programmes anyhow ... and we love doing that, don't we (16-C).

One participant described her experience as 'going on a holiday':

> It's very, very good ... [inaudible] like goin' on holiday, kinda thing, an' it's a bit like Polzeath, 'cause, you got the sea, the sea there [gestures], you got the boat there [gestures] and the houses there, and the sand, and there's people around you (05-ML).

Many participants commented on the people and animals, and appreciated the busy beach 'activity':

> Oh wow I can see a beach now. Oh yeah, it's a bit like Polzeath it is, with people on it. Oh yeah, people playing games an' that on the beach. It's hot 'cause they got their shorts and t-shirts on. It's very nice. Oh I can see a pink bucket as well. A ... a very busy beach ... very busy ... oh yeah, very nice. [inaudible] they're going out in the boat now. Oh yeah, there's a chap going out on the beach—on the boat now. Ooh, very nice (05-ML).

Another participant declared that she felt inspired to visit the places depicted in the VR nature experience ("Oh, inspired! [laughs]. I want to go and visit the places" [11-C]).

3.5. Strange and Scary: The VR Nature Experience Is Not Always Positive

There were some negative responses to the VR nature experience, finding them potentially confusing or strange, such as this carer:

> Well from what I saw of the little bits, when she [her Mother] was at the beach, she obviously quite liked that. I think under the water was a bit confusing for her." (07-C)

One participant said "Yeah, it's quite strange actually, 'cause it's not *quite* real. It's got a strange light to it. Sort of, edges on the figures and things" (12-ML), and at one point found it frightening:

> 12-ML: Back to the beach. Ooh, clouds. Oh the little group in the corner there . . . Ooh yeah.
>
> It's a lot better down here than when we were there and I was up the top, terrified . . . Ooh, I don't like this.
>
> Researcher: What is it?
>
> 12-ML: It's all steep and falling away into the sea below me. I'm sitting on a rock.
>
> Researcher: Are you OK, do you want to take it off?
>
> 12-ML: No.

3.6. Responses to VR Equipment

Some participants found the VR technology amazing, describing it as 'incredible', 'brilliant', 'clever' and 'remarkable'.

> Now it's gone right behind me. My neck won't swivel that far. How on earth do they do this? Oh gosh it makes it look so good that I want to go in the sea. Extraordinary marks in the sand. Absolutely amazing [inaudible] (02-C).

> Oh wow yeah. It's quite an amazing sort of thing. It's almost like an experience without the smells [laughs] (04-V).

However, many of the participants discussed issues with the equipment which included their confidence in using the equipment, its heaviness, difficulties with body movement, and with focus while wearing glasses.

Only a few of the participants claimed that they experienced no discomfort with the VR equipment. Some participants with dementia were uncomfortable with the headset; one removed it after 40 seconds (07-ML) and another commented when fitting the headset: "It's a bit heavy" (05-ML). This was echoed by a number of other participants and some said they would prefer something less 'intrusive' and more 'user-friendly' (07-C), that "actually sat on your head properly" (19-ML). Most agreed that they could only tolerate the headset for a short time (" . . . I think if you were to watch it for, if you watched a film on it for half an hour, or an hour, it would become a bit heavy then" (09-V). One participant suggested it could make the wearer feel nauseous:

> I could see that it could make you feel a bit queasy if you stayed in it for a long time. I think if it, it's made smaller and more comfortable, then it would be beneficial (12-ML).

A few of the participants commented that they had problems with body movement and could not turn round to see everything:

> the only problem was I wanted to be able to go round 180 degrees and I couldn't. I think a wheelie chair would be a terrific advantage because I think a lot of people aren't as mobile as I am, you know (02-C).

> That looked round a bit too hard for my neck (19-ML).

Some participants who wore glasses had problems with focus: ("perhaps I should have had it with me glasses on because it would have been a bit more focussed [11-V]); and one felt that her experience was spoiled:

> I found the first bit on the beach was quite blurred. I don't ... was that my eyes or was it? ... I was having quite a job focussing on a lot of that ... It just kind of spoilt, spoilt it for me a bit, because I couldn't see some of the detail in anything (14-V).

One of the participants with dementia described a strange light around the "edges on the figures and things" and that people had looked "not quite real" and were a "bit too brightly coloured" (12-ML).

A small number of the participants living with dementia noted that they would not be able to operate the VR technology without help. One participant wondered if the researcher would always be available to help:

> I mean you put it on and took it off. Will you always be there to put it on and take it off? (03-ML)

In contrast, a few felt confident that they would be able to use the VR equipment ("It's just pressing a couple of buttons" [19-ML]).

None of the participants living with dementia claimed to be using much technology in their daily lives ("Too old in the tooth for that!" [laughs] [08-ML]). One indicated that he had the expertise—a telecoms degree—but as his carer explained:

> You used to use all these things but you don't get along with it any more. I'm the one with the computer now. And mobile phone. You don't telephone out. You barely turn on the telly unless I do it and find the channel [both laugh] (03-C).

For another couple without a computer, the carer explained, "We're not interested. It isn't our era if you know what I mean" (16-C). Other carers described technology—such as smart phones, tablets and computers—used in their everyday lives:

> I've got my phone and my ipad, that sort of thing. And I get 'round it alright. But I'm not expert in it. But you know, if I want to find out something, I usually can do it some way or another. Or phone up me brother in Australia and ask him [laughs] (11-C).

Café volunteers believed that they could use the VR technology ("I'm not high-tech like you youngsters but I'm not illiterate either [laughs], so yes, I think I could do it" [14-V]) but were unsure if older carers, or people with dementia, would be able to use it:

> Maybe, maybe they would need someone with them all the time, if they didn't, to set it up for them. 'Cause I'm just thinking of how my husband was, and he wouldn't have been able to do that. Because unfortunately, I mean, he would always put music on for us for Saturday night while we had a nice meal. And then one night he said, well, he said 'I can't get the CD to play' and I said 'well you just press that button'. You see, it had just gone out of his mind. He, well, he lost his sort of, spatial awareness, thing. (18-V)

3.7. Volunteer Staff and Carers' Perceptions of VR for People with Dementia in Long Term Care

Generally, volunteer staff and carers felt that the VR nature experience was a 'good idea' for people with dementia in long term care settings. The perceived benefits included, accessing nature in an alternative way, relieving boredom, triggering memories, and improving mood and calming. However, they also had reservations, fearing that the person with dementia could find the VR experience potentially confusing and unable to cope with the equipment. Table 2 provides a summary of volunteer staff and carers' perceptions of VR for people with dementia in long term care.

4. Discussion

The purpose of this study was to explore the acceptability of VR nature environments for people with memory loss at memory cafes, and volunteer staff and carers' perceptions of VR for people with dementia in long-term care. The findings identified six themes around experiences and perceptions of the VR nature environment intervention. The VR experience was positive for participants, with a reported sensation of 'presence', the feeling of 'being there' on the beach or underwater as depicted in the VR scenes. That feeling of 'being there' whilst knowing that 'you are not actually there' has been referred to as 'place illusion' and it is this illusion that creates the 'wow' factor (p. 38, [10]). For some participants, the feeling of being transported to, for example, a local beach, evoked a sense of wonder and amazement. There is no sense of presence in physical reality [10], a notion that was captured well by the participant who contrasted the VR nature experience with the beautiful nature views from her home. Where participants responded to the events and people on the beaches as if they were real, they experienced the illusion that Slater and Sanchez-Vives (p. 5, [10]) refer to as 'plausibility'. Participants described how they felt that individuals on the beach were looking at them and might even talk with them, provoking their desire to interact, and indicating that they found the environment 'sufficiently credible'. These findings suggest that, for some of the participants, the VR nature environments intervention delivered an experience that generated an "illusory sense of place and an illusory sense of reality" (p. 5, [10]).

These findings support those from existing studies which found that people with dementia are able to perceive a sense of presence [22]. However, the sense of presence was not positive for all. With participants responding realistically to VR, it is hardly surprising that one participant reacted to her experience of 'sitting on a rock' with fear. This clearly affected her enjoyment and it is crucial to avoid participants feeling fear and anxiety, filming scenes that are sensitive to participants' needs. Whether the people with memory loss perceived a sense of presence was likely affected by the extent of their engagement with the VR experience, and the degree of their cognitive impairment; the more advanced their impairment, the greater the possibility they may have found it 'confusing' [6].

Participants reported not only the perception of 'being there' but also the feeling of 'being away', a key factor in Attention Restoration Theory [18] which posits that nature distracts from the everyday and mundane. 'Being away' had a dual perspective; one was experiencing familiar places that were no longer easily accessed, and the other was experiencing new places such as 'going on holiday' or 'going somewhere'. The familiarity of the VR nature scenes gave enjoyment to participants as they sought to identify exact locations and to relate stories and memories, often linked to particular places. By interacting with each other—the person with memory loss and the carer—participants were often able to create meaning around the 'virtual' places and connect them to their own personal lives. Arguably, this 'place-based reminiscence' helped participants to "re-experience past places" (p. 5, [23]). Such reminiscence could invoke joyful memories such as seaside holidays with children, but there could be a poignancy too, as participants reflected on how places were no longer accessible to them, usually because of transport and mobility issues. The potential of the VR nature experience to stimulate reminiscence could help people with dementia maintain continuity of the self [23,24] particularly important for people with dementia living in long term care who may feel this is broken.

VR nature also offered participants the opportunity to experience new places, or nature in a 'new' or different way. Participants found the scenes inviting them—to swim in the sea and to come away on a holiday, and perhaps, if neither of these were realistic options, then the virtual experience was an acceptable alternative. The scenes with the underwater coral reefs elicited a feeling of 'going somewhere', somewhere very different for the participant who had never been a good swimmer but who would have liked to explore 'under the sea' and never had the opportunity. Thus the VR nature experience gave such participants " . . . the possibility to step outside the normal bounds of reality and realise goals in a totally new and unexpected way" (p. 2, [10]).

The beauty of the nature scenes, with views of beaches and the sea, was highlighted by all, and was key to their engagement and enjoyment. Whilst immersed and contemplating the beauty of nature, some participants noted a calming and soothing effect, suggesting that virtual nature can induce a restorative experience. Brown, Mitchell [25] argue that a sense of wellbeing—which can reduce stress—should be the main ambition for meaningful activity in advanced dementia, and call for creative and innovative interventions that can improve quality of life for people with advanced dementia. Arguably, the VR nature environments shows promise for providing a 'stimulating' yet 'familiar environment' that engages people with dementia in a 'unique way' (p. 2, [9]).

5. Limitations

One limitation in this study was that the environment in the memory cafes was 'not ideal'; the VR nature experience was set up in a room where other activities were taking place and background noise could be a distraction for participants, as was the case with one participant who observed she would have liked to have heard the sounds of nature such as the 'roar of the sea'. Anderson, Mayer [26] noted the importance of reducing distraction from background noise when using VR but arguably, it could be challenging to be free of background noise in an aged-care environment.

Another potential limitation is that the VR world is a fast moving one and equipment and types of simulation are rapidly changing and developing; Sayma, Tuijt [9] found that differences in software and hardware availability could 'dramatically alter' the experience of participants in studies that were just one year apart. Since completion of this study, light-weighted headsets have been released and used successfully with participants with mild cognitive impairment [27]. Recent, and no doubt future, developments will make CGI immersion more straightforward for use with various populations. Financial constraints also impacted decisions on technology; for example, participants were unable to interact with the VR nature environments as we could not readily combine photorealism and interactivity within the budget constraints of the study.

6. Implications

The findings suggest that the VR natural environments intervention did engage a number of the participants. The researcher facilitated engagement, often with the help of a carer, so it is likely that for people living in long-term care, staff facilitation would be a requirement [6,22]. Similarly, it is unlikely that people with more advanced dementia would be able to use the technology without support from staff and carers [23]. The need for one-to-one support would be time-consuming for care home staff, causing some in the study to doubt if it is practical to introduce this technology into care homes for individuals with more severe dementia [16]. Future work should focus on the feasibility of implementing the VR nature experience in long-term care settings and should include assessing time consumption for one-to-one interaction and training requirements for care home staff. In future research, it would also be beneficial to understand the extent of study participants' cognitive impairment via standardised tests.

Perhaps the key issues for the technology of the VR nature experience were practical; many participants experienced discomfort with the headset, and as already noted, this is an area where technology improvements are ongoing [27]. However, issues with the HMD may mean that the VR nature environments intervention is 'not for everyone'. A few participants reported visual issues and, as people with dementia may have visuo-perception problems, this should be taken into account in future development. The experience was also limited for a few participants by being unable to turn through 360 degrees in their chair which could be addressed by using a 360° swivel armchair.

7. Conclusions

This study shows that people living with mild to moderate cognitive impairment who participated in a VR nature intervention had a sense of presence in the nature environments.

Despite the importance of presence in VR being recognised [28], few studies on immersive VR in dementia have attempted to establish participant presence [9]. Given that presence is a subjective experience, the qualitative approach used in this study contributes to a developing field of research where evidence is still limited. It also enhances our understanding of the wellbeing benefits that people with mild to moderate memory loss can derive from a VR nature intervention, and shows promise for those living in long-term care. Since people with advanced dementia in residential care are less involved in activities [29,30], the VR nature intervention could be a way of engaging them in meaningful activity—with support from carers. Future work should build on lessons learned from this study and continue to work with people with dementia in developing and implementing VR technology in long-term care settings.

Supplementary Materials: The following are available online at https://www.mdpi.com/2308-3417/6/1/27/s1. Framework Analysis Thematic Charts.

Author Contributions: Conceptualization, S.G.D., R.G., M.P.W., N.L.Y.; methodology, S.G.D., R.G., N.O., M.P.W., N.L.Y.; validation, S.G.D., R.G., M.P.W.; formal analysis, N.O., R.G., N.L.Y.; investigation, N.L.Y.; writing—original draft preparation, N.O.; writing—review and editing, N.O., N.L.Y., S.G.D., M.P.W., R.G.; supervision, S.G.D., R.G., M.P.W. All authors have read and agreed to the published version of the manuscript.

Funding: This research was funded by The College of Medicine and Health, University of Exeter (which funded the second author's PhD); The Blue Health project which received funding from the European Union's Horizon 2020 Research and Innovation Programme under grant agreement no. 666773; and The National Institute for Health Research (NIHR) Collaboration for Leadership in Applied Health Research and Care South West Peninsula at the Royal Devon and Exeter NHS Foundation Trust. Views expressed are those of the authors and not necessarily those of the University of Exeter, European Union, NHS, the NIHR, or the Department of Health.

Institutional Review Board Statement: The study was conducted according to the guidelines of the Declaration of Helsinki, and approved by the Medical School Ethics Committee of the University of Exeter (Jan19/B/192; January 2019).

Informed Consent Statement: Informed consent was obtained from all participants involved in the study.

Data Availability Statement: The data presented in this study are available in the supplementary material.

Acknowledgments: The authors would like to thank the Cornwall Memory Café Network for facilitating our access to the memory cafes, and all the café volunteers and visitors for agreeing to host the research; the participants themselves; the Minack Theatre for permission to film on their site; Alex Smalley for assistance with creating the 360° video; Chris Campkin for help with filming and editing; and the BBC's Natural History Unit, for permitting use of the Blue Planet II footage to help create the 360° video.

Conflicts of Interest: The authors declare no conflict of interest.

References

1. White, M.P.; Alcock, I.; Grellier, J.; Wheeler, B.W.; Hartig, T.; Warber, S.L.; Bone, A.; Depledge, M.H.; Fleming, L.E. Spending at least 120 minutes a week in nature is associated with good health and wellbeing. *Sci. Rep.* **2019**, *9*, 7730. [CrossRef]
2. Orr, N.; Wagstaffe, A.; Briscoe, S.; Garside, R. How do older people describe their sensory experiences of the natural world? A systematic review of the qualitative evidence. *BMC Geriatr.* **2016**, *16*, 116. [CrossRef]
3. NICE. Mental Wellbeing of Older People in Care Homes. In *Quality Standard QS50*; 2013; Available online: https://www.nice.org.uk/guidance/qs50 (accessed on 1 September 2020).
4. White, P.C.L.; Wyatt, J.; Chalfont, G.; Bland, J.M.; Neale, C.; Trepel, D.; Graham, H. Exposure to nature gardens has time-dependent associations with mood improvements for people with mid-and late-stage dementia: Innovative practice. *Dementia* **2018**, *17*, 627–634. [CrossRef] [PubMed]
5. Yeo, N.L.; Elliott, L.R.; Bethel, A.; White, M.P.; Dean, S.G.; Garside, R. Indoor nature interventions for health and wellbeing of older adults in residential settings: A systematic review. *Gerontologist* **2020**, *60*, e184–e199. [CrossRef]

6. Moyle, W.; Jones, C.; Dwan, T.; Petrovich, T. Effectiveness of a virtual reality forest on people with dementia: A mixed methods pilot study. *Gerontologist* **2018**, *58*, 478–487. [CrossRef] [PubMed]
7. Reynolds, L.; Rodiek, S.; Lininger, M.; McCulley, M.A. Can a virtual nature experience reduce anxiety and agitation in people with dementia? *J. Hous. Elder.* **2018**, *32*, 176–193. [CrossRef]
8. Yeo, N.L.; White, M.P.; Alcock, I.; Garside, R.; Dean, S.G.; Smalley, A.J.; Gatersleben, B. What is the best way of delivering virtual nature for improving mood? An experimental comparison of high definition TV, 360° video, and computer generated virtual reality. *J. Environ. Psychol.* **2020**, *72*, 101500. [CrossRef] [PubMed]
9. Sayma, M.; Tuijt, R.; Cooper, C.; Walters, K. Are We There Yet? Immersive Virtual Reality to Improve Cognitive Function in Dementia and Mild Cognitive Impairment. *Gerontologist* **2020**, *60*, e502–e512. [CrossRef]
10. Slater, M.; Sanchez-Vives, M.V. Enhancing our lives with immersive virtual reality. *Front. Robot. AI* **2016**, *3*, 74. [CrossRef]
11. Heim, M. The design of virtual reality. *Body Soc.* **1995**, *1*, 65–77. [CrossRef]
12. Murray, C. Towards a phenomenology of the body in virtual reality. *Res. Philos. Technol.* **1999**, *19*, 149–173.
13. Low, K.E. The social life of the senses: Charting directions. *Sociol. Compass* **2012**, *6*, 271–282. [CrossRef]
14. Slater, M. Place illusion and plausibility can lead to realistic behaviour in immersive virtual environments. *Philos. Trans. R. Soc. B Biol. Sci.* **2009**, *364*, 3549–3557. [CrossRef]
15. Mitzner, T.L.; Boron, J.B.; Fausset, C.B.; Adams, A.E.; Charness, N.; Czaja, S.J.; Dijkstra, K.; Fisk, A.D.; Rogers, W.A.; Sharit, J. Older adults talk technology: Technology usage and attitudes. *Comput. Hum. Behav.* **2010**, *26*, 1710–1721. [CrossRef]
16. Goodall, G.; Taraldsen, K.; Serrano, J.A. The use of technology in creating individualized, meaningful activities for people living with dementia: A systematic review. *Dementia* **2020**. [CrossRef] [PubMed]
17. Sekhon, M.; Cartwright, M.; Francis, J.J. Acceptability of healthcare interventions: An overview of reviews and development of a theoretical framework. *BMC Health Serv. Res.* **2017**, *17*, 88. [CrossRef] [PubMed]
18. Kaplan, R.K.S. *The Experience of Nature: A Psychological Perspective*; Cambridge University Press: Cambridge, UK, 1989.
19. Cohen-Mansfield, J.; Dakheel-Ali, M.; Marx, M.S. Engagement in persons with dementia: The concept and its measurement. *Am. J. Geriatr. Psychiatry* **2009**, *17*, 299–307. [CrossRef] [PubMed]
20. Ritchie, J.L.J. *Qualitative Research Practice: A Guide for Social Science Students and Researchers*; Sage: London, UK, 2003.
21. Gale, N.K.; Heath, G.; Cameron, E.; Rashid, S.; Redwood, S. Using the framework method for the analysis of qualitative data in multi-disciplinary health research. *BMC Med. Res. Methodol.* **2013**, *13*, 117. [CrossRef]
22. Flynn, D.; Van Schaik, P.; Blackman, T.; Femcott, C.; Hobbs, B.; Calderon, C. Developing a virtual reality—Based methodology for people with dementia: A feasibility study. *Cyber Psychol. Behav.* **2003**, *6*, 591–611. [CrossRef] [PubMed]
23. Siriaraya, P.; Ang, C.S. Recreating living experiences from past memories through virtual worlds for people with dementia. In Proceedings of the SIGCHI Conference on Human Factors in Computing Systems, Toronto, ON, Canada, 26 April 2014.
24. Bluck, S. Autobiographical memory: Exploring its functions in everyday life. *Memory* **2003**, *11*, 113–123. [CrossRef]
25. Brown, M.; Mitchell, B.; Boyd, A.; Tolson, D. Meaningful activity in advanced dementia. *Nurs. Older People* **2020**, *32*. [CrossRef]
26. Anderson, A.P.; Mayer, M.D.; Fellows, A.M.; Cowan, D.R.; Hegel, M.T.; Buckey, J.C. Relaxation with immersive natural scenes presented using virtual reality. *Aerosp. Med. Hum. Perform.* **2017**, *88*, 520–526. [CrossRef] [PubMed]
27. Park, J.-H.; Liao, Y.; Kim, D.-R.; Song, S.; Lim, J.H.; Park, H.; Lee, Y.; Park, K.W. Feasibility and tolerability of a culture-based virtual reality (VR) training program in patients with mild cognitive impairment: A randomized controlled pilot study. *Int. J. Environ. Res. Public Health* **2020**, *17*, 3030. [CrossRef] [PubMed]
28. Garrett, B.; Taverner, T.; Gromala, D.; Tao, G.; Cordingley, E.; Sun, C. Virtual reality clinical research: Promises and challenges. *JMIR Serious Games* **2018**, *6*, e10839. [CrossRef]
29. Smit, D.; De Lange, J.; Willemse, B.; Twisk, J.; Pot, A.M. Activity involvement and quality of life of people at different stages of dementia in long term care facilities. *Aging Ment. Health* **2016**, *20*, 100–109. [CrossRef]
30. Smith, N.; Towers, A.-M.; Palmer, S.; Beecham, J.; Welch, E. Being occupied: Supporting 'meaningful activity' in care homes for older people in England. *Ageing Soc.* **2018**, *38*, 2218–2240. [CrossRef]

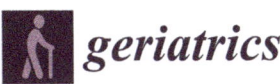

Communication

Feasibility of a Small Group Otago Exercise Program for Older Adults Living with Dementia

Julie D. Ries * and Martha Carroll

Center for Optimal Aging, Physical Therapy Department, School of Health Sciences,
College of Health & Education, Marymount University, Arlington, VA 22207, USA; mcarroll@marymount.edu
* Correspondence: jries@marymount.edu

Abstract: Older adults with dementia experience more frequent and injurious falls than their cognitively-intact peers; however, there are no evidence-based fall-prevention programs (EBFPP) for this population. The Otago Exercise Program (OEP) is an EBFPP for older adults that has not been well-studied in people with dementia. We sought to explore the feasibility of group delivery of OEP in an adult day health center (ADHC) for people with dementia. We collected demographic data, Functional Assessment Staging Tool (FAST), and Mini Mental State Exam (MMSE) scores for seven participants with dementia. Pre- and post-test data included: Timed-Up-and-Go (TUG), 30-Second Chair-Stand (30s-CST), Four-Stage-Balance-Test (4-SBT), and Berg Balance Scale (BBS). We implemented a supervised group OEP, 3x/week × 8 weeks. Most participants required 1:1 supervision for optimal challenge and participation. Five participants completed the program. All had moderately severe to severe dementia based upon FAST; MMSE scores ranged from mild to severe cognitive impairment. Four of five participants crossed the threshold from higher to lower fall risk in at least one outcome (TUG, 30s-CST, 4-SBT, or BBS), and four of five participants improved by >Minimal Detectable Change (MDC_{90}) score in at least one outcome. The group delivery format of OEP required significant staff oversight for optimal participation, making the program unsustainable.

Keywords: dementia; balance; falls; exercise; Otago Exercise Program

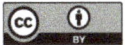

1. Introduction

Exercise alone, or as a component of a comprehensive fall-prevention program, can effectively decrease falls in older adults [1–4]. There is cautious optimism for exercise interventions to reduce falls in individuals with dementia (IwD) [5], but there are no identified evidence-based fall-prevention programs (EBFPPs) for this population [4,6,7]. IwD display an increased prevalence and frequency of falls, and are more likely to be seriously injured from a fall than their cognitively-intact age-matched peers [8–10]. The Otago Exercise Program (OEP) [11], comprised of strength and balance exercises and a walking program, is one of the EBFPPs supported by the STEADI (Stopping Elderly Accidents, Deaths, and Injuries) initiative of the US Center for Disease Control and Prevention (CDC) [12]. The OEP has not been well-studied with IwD. Suttanon et al. [13] found an in-home OEP-based program to be feasible and safe for participants with mild to moderate Alzheimer disease (MMSE mean score 21/30). A retrospective study by Trappuzano et al. [14] showed some benefit of home health administered OEP for people with dementia (miniCog mean score of 1.76/5), and Beato et al. [15] and Knott et al. [16] retrospectively found a positive impact of an OEP-based intervention for assisted-living residents without commenting on the cognitive status of participants.

Group administration of OEP is beginning to be represented in the literature. Kocic et al. [17] provided OEP in a nursing home setting, where two physiotherapists oversaw groups of up to ten participants, but they intentionally excluded those with cognitive impairment. Renfro et al. [18] demonstrated the feasibility of a community-based group OEP with adults with intellectual disabilities. In long-term care, Kovàcs et al. [19] compared group OEP to no exercise for older adults with cognitive impairment (mean MMSE 21/30) and demonstrated improvements in balance, but not falls, in the OEP group. Any enthusiasm for "group" OEP is quelled with careful reading of these studies: Renfro et al. averaged classes of 8 participants with the help of "2–3 caregivers/staff, 5–7 nursing students, and 1 or 2 PI/PTs" [18] (p. 4) (it appears there may have been days where the help outnumbered the participants!), and Kovàcs et al. delivered the program with two physiotherapists for groups of 2–4 participants [19]. Recently, a series of studies in nursing home settings has supported the feasibility of group OEP with residents with physical and cognitive frailty [20–23]. While the mean MMSE scores of participants represent cognitive impairment (21–22/30) [20,21], a diagnosis of dementia was not in the inclusion criteria of any of these studies. The strategy for group administration of OEP in two of these studies was to initiate the program in small groups (6 participants to 3 staff [21] or 4–7 participants to 1 staff [22]) and after 4 weeks, to combine all small groups into one larger group with 3 staff providing oversight to groups of 18 and 29, respectively. The mechanics of group OEP administration in the other studies (i.e., size of group and number of staff) was not presented [20,23].

The purpose of this communication is to share findings of a small feasibility study for group OEP for IwD at an Adult Day Health Center (ADHC) and, secondarily, to provide insights on group exercise for IwD. Most ADHC settings provide seated group exercise activities, but not standing/upright exercises, as staff must cater to the lowest level of functioning for safety and maximal participation. There is benefit to physical therapist (PT)-directed exercise programs in improving balance in participants of ADHC [24,25], but we are striving for a program that can be sustained with consultation from, rather than direct oversight by, a PT.

OEP [11,26] starts with a series of five warm-up/flexibility exercises for the head/neck, trunk, and ankles. Strength-training exercises include seated knee extension, ankle dorsiflexion and plantar flexion, and standing knee flexion and hip abduction. Cuff weights provide resistance and are increased when the participant completes 2 sets of 10 repetitions without complaint. Balance exercises are performed in an upright position (standing or walking) and are progressed by decreasing upper extremity (UE) support. They include partial squats, sit to stand, sideways walking, backward walking, walking with turns, single limb stance, tandem stance, heel-toe walking, walking on heels, walking on toes, backward heel–toe walking, and stair climbing (we omitted stair climbing as we did not have easy access to stairs).

OEP is imperfect as a comprehensive balance training program as it is solely driven by anticipatory balance challenges of base-of-support/center-of-gravity manipulation. We were willing to forego balance training with a more robust design (i.e., inclusive of changing visual (eyes closed, scanning environment) and somatosensory experience (walking and balancing on foam and other altered surfaces), reactive challenges (perturbations, prop use), deliberate dual tasking (superimposing cognitive and physical tasks)), in exchange for a program transferrable to ADHC oversight. The prescriptive nature of OEP, replete with manual and pictures, was considered an asset of the program.

2. Materials and Methods

This exploratory study is categorized as an "intervention development" feasibility study [27], a preliminary step to determine if a formal feasibility study of group OEP that can be sustained by ADHC staff is realistic and appropriate. The study was approved by the Marymount University Institutional Review Board (MUIRB#387) and written informed consent was provided by legal proxy decision-makers.

A sample of convenience of seven individuals at a local county-sponsored ADHC met the inclusion criteria of: physician diagnosis of dementia, medical stability, ability to walk without physical assistance (assistive device acceptable), and ability to follow one-step commands. Exclusion criteria included: unstable or limiting systemic pathology;

any surgery or cancer diagnosis or treatment within previous six months. Demographic data, collected from facility health records, are presented in Table 1. Mini-Mental Status Examination (MMSE) [28] and the Functional Assessment Staging Tool (FAST) [29] were administered by the facility nurse. A score of ≤23 on the MMSE is the generally accepted indicator of cognitive impairment, with 18 to 23 indicating mild impairment and 0 to 17 indicating more severe impairment [30]. The FAST reveals functional implications of dementia on daily life.

Table 1. Participant characteristics.

	Participants							Mean/Median All Participants $n = 7$	Mean/Median Completers $n = 5$
	1	2	3	4	5	6	7		
Sex	M	F	F	M	F	F	F	71% Female	60% Female
Age (years)	85	89	90	72	89	79	83	83.9	85
MMSE Score	17/30	20/30	6/30	24/30	14/30	22/30	20/30	Mean = 17.6 Median = 20	Mean = 16.2 Median = 17
FAST Score	6A	6B	7A	6C	6A	6D	6C	Median = 6	Median = 6
Comorbidities	8 (a [3], b [2], f, g [2])	6 (a [2], b, d, h [2])	5 (a [2], d [2], d)	4 (a, c, e, g)	4 (a [3], g)	5 (a [2], b, c, e)	7 (a [2], b, c, d, e, f)	5.6	5.4
Medications	5	5	6	7	4	6	6	5.6	5.4
Fall in Past Year	No	Yes	Yes	Yes	No	Yes	No	N/A	N/A
Assistive Device	None	RW	None	None	None	Cane	RW	N/A	N/A
Attendance	96%	96%	65%	74%	96%	0	0	N/A	85.4%

MMSE = Mini Mental Status Exam; FAST = Functional Assessment Staging Tool (A through D represent progressive levels of impairment); RW = rolling walker. Comorbidities: a = cardiovascular disease (e.g., hypertension, hypercholesterolemia, atrial fibrillation, orthostatic hypotension, syncope); b = endocrine/thyroid disorder (e.g., diabetes, hypothyroid); c = neuro disorder (e.g., Parkinson's disease, stroke, seizure disorder); d = ortho disorder (e.g., osteoporosis, arthritis); e = psychological/psychiatric disorder (e.g., anxiety, depression); f = vision disorder (e.g., cataracts, macular degeneration); g = gastrointestinal/genitourinary disorder (e.g., GERD, chronic constipation, kidney disease); h = history of cancer.

Measures of balance and gait were assessed within two weeks prior to, and one week following, the intervention. Informed by the STEADI initiative [31], we administered: Timed Up-and-Go (TUG), 30 s Chair Stand Test (30s-CST), and 4-Stage Balance Test (4-SBT). Additionally, participants performed the Berg Balance Scale (BBS). Tests were performed in the order presented below and were scored onsite by the tester and scored on video by a second PT. On the rare occasion that scores were not corroborated, the therapists came to consensus on the final score.

For the TUG [32], participants began seated in a chair with arm rests, were instructed to walk "quickly, but safely", and on the instruction "Go", stood, walked 3 m, circled around a cone, walked back to the chair, and sat down. As has been previously documented [33], timing began with movement initiation as opposed to the "Go" command and finished when the buttocks contacted the chair. Cuing was provided as needed (e.g., "go around the cone", "sit in that chair"). The score was the mean time of two trials. The OEP Manual [34] suggests that the cutoff score of ≥12 s indicates a higher risk of falls, consistent with evidence by Lusardi et al. [35].

The 30s-CST [36] is the number of stands completed in 30 s without the use of arms. A 17-inch seat-to-floor height chair was used, and cuing was offered throughout the test as needed, encouraging continued efforts [37]. The OEP Manual [34] suggests individuals performing below age and sex-matched norms are at higher risk of falls, consistent with evidence that LE strength is associated with fall risk [4].

The 4-SBT requires balancing in each of 4 foot positions for 10 s (feet together, semi-tandem, tandem, single-limb stance) and is based on the FICSIT-4 (Frailty and Injuries: Cooperative Studies of Intervention Techniques) [38], which uses the same foot positions with more complex scoring. There is some precedent for use of the 4-SBT [14] and FIC-

SIT [39,40] in dementia research. Evidence that community living older adults unable to maintain tandem stance ≥10 s are at higher risk of falls [41] makes the inability to sustain position 3 (tandem) an indication of fall risk in the OEP Manual [34].

The BBS consists of 14 progressively challenging, functionally oriented balance activities, ranging in difficulty from sitting unsupported to turning in a circle and single-limb stance. Each item is scored from 0 (unable to perform) to 4 (proficient performance). The BBS has been used with older adults with cognitive impairment [42,43]. Lusardi et al. [35] identify <50 as a cutoff score for fall risk in community-dwelling older adults.

The exercise intervention was an 8 week, 3x/week, 45 min class following the OEP curriculum [11,26]. The PTs overseeing exercise classes completed online OEP instructor training [26] and were well-versed in OEP administration and program fidelity; student instructors were trained by these PTs. All instructors were trained in communication and rehabilitation principles to facilitate optimal success with IwD [44]. The program was performed in the therapy room of the ADHC at a consistent time with a consistent PT instructor, occasional support of a second PT, and student instructors (nursing and PT students). Music, chosen by participants, was played during the class. The goal was to have one instructor oversee as many participants as possible, providing it was safe and effective. Based on our experience in this venue, we planned to oversee a class of 9 participants with 3 instructors; with 5 participants, we envisioned 2 instructors would suffice. It quickly became apparent that optimal engagement (i.e., participants consistently performing exercises at a level of appropriate challenge) would require closer oversight. Initially, when we attempted to run classes with fewer instructors, the time/repetition per task and intensity of challenge all suffered. It was never unsafe, just ineffective. Without a "personal instructor", attention waned and the tendency for self-challenge was feeble in all but one participant (Participant 1). Ultimately, we used at most 1:2, but usually 1:1 supervision. The staff of the ADHC oversaw the walking component of the program and charted participation.

3. Results

While participants sometimes exercised during our class without 1:1 supervision, they rarely challenged themselves or sustained the activity independently. When participants were not maximally engaged, student instructors stepped in to assist, which inevitably enhanced participation. We made efforts to wane supervision repeatedly throughout the 8 week intervention, but this resulted in reversion to less effort and/or attention from participants. Prioritizing safety, we had 1:1 supervision with our most physically impaired participants who were at highest risk for falls (Participants 2 and 4). Participants 3 and 5 required constant and focused supervision to remain cognitively engaged. Participant 1 was the only participant who did not require constant 1:1 supervision for optimal participation; thus, he was usually paired with Participant 2 (staff could provide physical assistance to Participant 2 and verbal cuing to Participant 1).

Seven participants underwent pre-testing and two withdrew prior to the intervention due to unrelated medical issues. The withdrawn participants were slightly younger and slightly higher in MMSE scores, as evidenced in comparing means/median scores of all participants ($n = 7$) vs. only those who completed the intervention ($n = 5$) (Table 1). All participants, save one, rated FAST Stage 6 ("moderately severe dementia"), demonstrating difficulty with the pragmatics of dressing, bathing, and toileting. Participant 3 was rated Stage 7 ("severe dementia"), as evidenced by a dependency on ADLs and minimally preserved speech. Participant data were analyzed by comparing changes in pre- and post-test performance with established Minimal Detectable Change scores at the 90% confidence interval (MDC_{90}) for older adults with dementia. A change score exceeding the MDC_{90} score is thought to represent a "true" change (i.e., beyond what would be expected from individual variability and/or measurement error). The MDC_{90} score used for the TUG was 4.09 s [33]; for the 30s-CST, it was 2 repetitions [37]; and for the BBS, it was 6.4 [45]. While the 4-SBT has been used in dementia research, the published MDC_{95} score for this population of 1.5 units was based on the FICSIT scoring model, and therefore does not translate to 4-SBT [40]. In determining outcomes related to 4-SBT, we focused on position 3 (tandem stance) as a cutoff score and looked for changes in performance from <3 to ≥3 to represent a clinically meaningful change.

Outcomes are presented in Table 2. One participant (Participant 3) improved TUG performance by >MDC_{90}, and four participants improved their 30s-CST by ≥MDC_{90}. Participants 3 and 4 not only improved by MDC_{90} but hit the threshold for age/sex matched norms for 30s-CST, indicating a transition from higher to lower fall risk. Participant 1 performed well above the norm for 30s-CST, and Participants 3 and 5 showed improvement within the norm spectrum. Three of the five participants who failed tandem stance in the 4-SBT pre-test passed the post-test, which in the context of fall risk is considered an important milestone [41]. There were no adverse events during testing or interventions. There were two reported non-injurious falls at home over the course of the study, both by Participant 2. Participant 4's spouse became an unofficial participant and official volunteer with the program over the course of the 8 week intervention.

Table 2. Participant outcomes.

	Participant 1			Participant 2			Participant 3			Participant 4			Participant 5		
	Pre-Test	Post-Test	Δ Score	Pre-Test	Post-Test	Δ Score	Pre-Test	Post-Test	Δ Score	Pre-Test	Post-Test	Δ Score	Pre-Test	Post-Test	Δ Score
TUG (sec)	10.5	11.6	(1.1)	48.5	46.1	2.4	25.0	17.6	7.4 [a]	11.3	9.4	1.9	13.5	14.8	(1.3)
30s-CST (reps)	16	20	4 [a]	0	0	0	6	9	3 [a]	9	15	6 [ab]	8	10	2 [a]
4-SBT	2	3	1 [b]	2	2	0	2	3	1 [b]	2	2	0	2	3	1 [b]
BBS	51	54	3	27	24	(3)	44	45	1	41	43	2	52	51	(1)
Supervision needs	• Paired with another participant (2) for oversight • Frequent verbal cuing required for optimal level of challenge			• Required 1:1 oversight • Constant physical assistance required for safety and optimal level of challenge			• Required 1:1 oversight • Constant physical assistance and verbal cuing required for safety and optimal level of challenge			• Required 1:1 oversight • Constant physical assistance and verbal cuing required for safety and optimal level of challenge			• Required 1:1 oversight • Constant physical presence and verbal cuing required for optimal level of challenge		

Δ Score = change score, TUG = Timed Up-And-Go, 30s-CST = 30-s Chair Stand Test, 4-SBT = 4 Stage Balance Test, BBS = Berg Balance Scale. Parenthetical numbers show negative change, none of which met MDC_{90} and therefore represent no "true" change in performance. [a] = Performance change meets minimal detectable change (MDC_{90}) score; shows true positive change (improved performance in post-test). [b] = Performance change represents change from higher to lower fall risk per OEP guidelines (i.e., from fail to pass Position 3 (tandem stance) in 4-SBT, from below to within age & sex matched norms for 30s-CST).

4. Discussion

The purpose of this preliminary study was to determine the feasibility of a group OEP for IwD that could be sustained by ADHC staff. In facilitating progress from a physiologic and motor learning standpoint, the importance of maximizing engagement and challenge for individual participants is an important consideration [46]. The need for four staff members to provide an optimal challenge and engagement of five participants was not sustainable. Maximizing the challenge did not appear to be a priority in recent published studies, which either do not comment on efforts to individualize the intervention [21,22] or allude to progressing the group as a whole [23]. Chen et al. [20] mention that physiotherapists "guided" participants to modify their exercise level, but the weights used were consistent at 0.5 kg and nurses "led" the intervention, so it is not clear how often physiotherapists may have guided these changes.

In comparison to other studies of group OEP administration [19–22], our participants were more cognitively impaired (diagnosis of dementia, mean MMSE of 16), and notably, the most physically impaired (forcing 1:1 supervision for safety) were the most cognitively capable. This contributed to our increased staff requirements. Existing studies, without commenting on efforts to maximize engagement and challenge of participants, identify beneficial outcomes of group OEP [20–23]. In reconsidering the feasibility of group administration of OEP, clear prioritization of safety over maximizing challenge may decrease the need for staff supervision.

One might assume that the need for such close supervision for optimal engagement negates the benefit of an exercise class (i.e., why not just work independently with participants?), but we perceived a strong social benefit from interactions within each class. A recent systematic review suggests that exercise administered in group format for IwD is associated with higher adherence rates [47]. An atmosphere of joy was a deliberate component of our intervention, and smiling, laughing, and joking were routine occurrences. Participants' music preferences drove the class playlist each day, creating the opportunity to hear and talk about personal favorites ranging from Latin instrumental to the Rolling Stones! Gonçalves et al. [48], in striving to establish core outcome measures, determined that the outcome most frequently sought by individuals with dementia and their caregivers was "enjoyment". Fun has been identified as a relevant characteristic of group exercise classes for fall prevention in older adults and, in fact, immediate enjoyment and social interaction may be more influential in motivating older adults to exercise than the promise of decreasing the fall risk [49]. Booth et al. [50], in a review of exercise-based fall-prevention programs, highlight the relevance of enjoyment in the context of motivating IwD, who may not be as self-actualized as their cognitively-intact peers. The benefit of a shared exercise experience is consistent with the findings of Lindelöf et al. [51], who, in a qualitative study of participants with dementia, found a theme of "Togetherness gives comfort, joy, and encouragement". A second theme in their study, "Exercise evokes body memories", was also represented in our study, as participants spoke of their younger life physical capabilities with pride and fondness. One participant reminisced about being a competitive track athlete, and another spoke of her days as a physical education teacher and coach. They were encouraged to tap into these memories throughout the class.

Over the course of the study, four of five participants crossed the threshold from higher to lower fall risk in at least one outcome, and four of five participants improved by >MDC_{90} change score in at least one outcome. Given the substantial methodological limitations of the small sample size and lack of control group, we cannot draw any conclusions about the impact of OEP. We did learn that our framework for bringing group OEP to ADHC is not feasible, as it is not sustainable. Our intent was to have the ADHC sustain the program, such that the dosage would reach recommended levels for older adults of >50 h over 6 months (i.e., 2 h/week), providing the best opportunity for fall reduction impact [52]. Instead, at the completion of this study, the OEP class participants rejoined the seated exercise group activity.

One consideration in sustaining balance training for this population is the benefit of educating and engaging caregivers, and working as a team (clinician, family/caregiver, patient/participant) to facilitate ongoing efforts. Meyer et al. [53] demonstrate that effective knowledge translation of fall-prevention strategies requires an inclusive approach that respects and understands the perspective of the person with dementia and their caregiver. The wife of Participant 4 was a regular ADHC volunteer and became an unofficial member of the class on her volunteer days. She was motivated by the experience to continue OEP with her husband at home when the study concluded and felt that she and her husband were both benefitting. Engaging dyads of IwD and care partners in OEP classes may be a future research direction.

5. Conclusions

The administration of a small group OEP 3x/week for 8 weeks with the prioritization of maximizing individual engagement and challenge was not feasible for ADHC sustainability. The perceived social benefit of group delivery encourages us to continue searching for sustainable group balance training options for ADHC participants.

Author Contributions: J.D.R. was responsible for the conceptualization, methodology, project administration, writing (original draft, review and editing), and funding acquisition. M.C. participated in project administration and writing (review and editing). All authors have read and agreed to the published version of the manuscript.

Funding: This research was partially funded by US Department of Health & Human Services, Administration for Community Living Grant: DHHS:ACL 90FPSG0012-01-00.

Institutional Review Board Statement: The study was conducted according to the guidelines of the Declaration of Helsinki, and approved by the Institutional Review Board of Marymount University (Protocol MUIRB#387).

Informed Consent Statement: Written informed consent was obtained from guardians who were established as decision makers for the Adult Day Health Center participants.

Data Availability Statement: Data for this pilot study are available from the corresponding author.

Acknowledgments: We are grateful to the wonderful participants, their families, and the staff of the ADHC, and for the commitment of a conscientious group of students/assistants: Nicole Dierkes, Gia Gossai, Shannon Gunning, Charlotte Hepler, Matthew Smith, and Becca Barnes.

Conflicts of Interest: The authors declare no conflict of interest.

References

1. Sherrington, C. Exercise for Preventing Falls in Older People Living in the Community. *Cochrane Database Syst. Rev.* **2019**, *1*, CD012424. [CrossRef] [PubMed]
2. Guirguis-Blake, J.M.; Michael, Y.L.; Perdue, L.A.; Coppola, E.L.; Beil, T.L. Interventions to Prevent Falls in Older Adults: Updated Evidence Report and Systematic Review for the US Preventive Services Task Force. *JAMA* **2018**, *319*, 1705–1716. [CrossRef]
3. Sherrington, C.; Fairhall, N.; Kwok, W.; Wallbank, G.; Tiedemann, A.; Michaleff, Z.A.; Ng, C.A.C.M.; Bauman, A. Evidence on Physical Activity and Falls Prevention for People Aged 65+ Years: Systematic Review to Inform the WHO Guidelines on Physical Activity and Sedentary Behaviour. *Int. J. Behav. Nutr. Phys. Act.* **2020**, *17*, 144. [CrossRef] [PubMed]
4. Panel on Prevention of Falls in Older Persons, American Geriatrics Society and British Geriatrics Society. Summary of the Updated American Geriatrics Society/British Geriatrics Society Clinical Practice Guideline for Prevention of Falls in Older Persons. *J. Am. Geriatr. Soc.* **2011**, *59*, 148–157. [CrossRef] [PubMed]
5. Burton, E.; Cavalheri, V.; Adams, R.; Browne, C.O.; Bovery-Spencer, P.; Fenton, A.M.; Campbell, B.W.; Hill, K.D. Effectiveness of Exercise Programs to Reduce Falls in Older People with Dementia Living in the Community: A Systematic Review and Meta-Analysis. *Clin. Interv. Aging* **2015**, *10*, 421–434. [CrossRef]
6. Lach, H.W.; Harrison, B.E.; Phongphanngam, S. Falls and Fall Prevention in Older Adults With Early-Stage Dementia: An Integrative Review. *Res. Gerontol. Nurs.* **2017**, *10*, 139–148. [CrossRef]
7. Peek, K.; Bryant, J.; Carey, M.; Dodd, N.; Freund, M.; Lawson, S.; Meyer, C. Reducing Falls among People Living with Dementia: A Systematic Review. *Dementia* **2018**, *19*, 1621–1640. [CrossRef]
8. Tinetti, M.E.; Speechley, M.; Ginter, S.F. Risk Factors for Falls among Elderly Persons Living in the Community. *N. Engl. J. Med.* **1988**, *319*, 1701–1707. [CrossRef]
9. Allali, G.; Launay, C.P.; Blumen, H.M.; Callisaya, M.L.; De Cock, A.-M.; Kressig, R.W.; Srikanth, V.; Steinmetz, J.-P.; Verghese, J.; Beauchet, O.; et al. Falls, Cognitive Impairment, and Gait Performance: Results From the GOOD Initiative. *J. Am. Med. Dir. Assoc.* **2016**, *18*, 335–340. [CrossRef]
10. Montero-Odasso, M.; Speechley, M. Falls in Cognitively Impaired Older Adults: Implications for Risk Assessment And Prevention. *J. Am. Geriatr. Soc.* **2018**, *66*, 367–375. [CrossRef]
11. Campbell, A.J.; Robertson, M.C. *Otago Exercise Programme to Prevent Falls in Older Adults*; Accident Compensation Corporation (ACC), Otago Medical School, University of Otago: Dunedin, New Zealand, 2003.
12. Kaniewski, M.; Stevens, J.A.; Parker, E.M.; Lee, R. An Introduction to the Centers for Disease Control and Prevention's Efforts to Prevent Older Adult Falls. *Front. Public Health* **2015**, *2*, 119. [CrossRef] [PubMed]
13. Suttanon, P.; Hill, K.D.; Said, C.M.; Williams, S.B.; Byrne, K.N.; Logiudice, D.; Lautenschlager, N.T.; Dodd, K.J. Feasibility, Safety and Preliminary Evidence of the Effectiveness of a Home-Based Exercise Programme for Older People with Alzheimer's Disease: A Pilot Randomized Controlled Trial. *Clin. Rehabil.* **2013**, *27*, 427–438. [CrossRef] [PubMed]
14. Trapuzzano, A.; McCarthy, L.; Dawson, N. Investigating the Effects of an Otago-Based Program among Individuals Living with Dementia. *Phys. Occup. Ther. Geriatr.* **2020**, *38*, 185–198. [CrossRef]
15. Beato, M.; Dawson, N.; Svien, L.; Wharton, T. Examining the Effects of an Otago-Based Home Exercise Program on Falls and Fall Risks in an Assisted Living Facility. *J. Geriatr. Phys. Ther.* **2018**, *42*, 224–229. [CrossRef] [PubMed]
16. Knott, S.; Hollis, A.; Jimenez, D.; Dawson, N.; Mabbagu, E.; Beato, M. Efficacy of Traditional Physical Therapy Versus Otago-Based Exercise in Fall Prevention for ALF-Residing Older Adults. *J. Geriatr. Phys. Ther.* **2021**, *44*, 210–218. [CrossRef] [PubMed]
17. Kocic, M.; Stojanovic, Z.; Nikolic, D.; Lazovic, M.; Grbic, R.; Dimitrijevic, L.; Milenkovic, M. The Effectiveness of Group Otago Exercise Program on Physical Function in Nursing Home Residents Older than 65 years: A Randomized Controlled Trial. *Arch. Gerontol. Geriatr.* **2018**, *75*, 112–118. [CrossRef]

18. Renfro, M.; Bainbridge, D.B.; Smith, M.L. Validation of Evidence-Based Fall Prevention Programs for Adults with Intellectual and/or Developmental Disorders: A Modified Otago Exercise Program. *Front. Public Health* **2016**, *4*, 261. [CrossRef]
19. Kovács, E.; Sztruhár Jónásné, I.; Karóczi, C.K.; Korpos, A.; Gondos, T. Effects of a Multimodal Exercise Program on Balance, Functional Mobility and Fall Risk in Older Adults with Cognitive Impairment: A Randomized Controlled Single-Blind Study. *Eur. J. Phys. Rehabil. Med.* **2013**, *49*, 639–648.
20. Chen, X.; Zhao, L.; Liu, Y.; Zhou, Z.; Zhang, H.; Wei, D.; Chen, J.; Li, Y.; Ou, J.; Huang, J.; et al. Otago Exercise Programme for Physical Function and Mental Health among Older Adults with Cognitive Frailty during COVID-19: A Randomised Controlled Trial. *J. Clin. Nurs.* **2021**, in press. [CrossRef]
21. Feng, H.; Zou, Z.; Zhang, Q.; Wang, L.; Ouyang, Y.-Q.; Chen, Z.; Ni, Z. The Effect of the Group-Based Otago Exercise Program on Frailty among Nursing Home Older Adults with Cognitive Impairment. *Geriatr. Nurs.* **2021**, *42*, 479–483. [CrossRef]
22. Zou, Z.; Chen, Z.; Ni, Z.; Hou, Y.; Zhang, Q. The Effect of Group-Based Otago Exercise Program on Fear of Falling and Physical Function among Older Adults Living in Nursing Homes: A Pilot Trial. *Geriatr. Nurs.* **2021**, *43*, 288–292. [CrossRef] [PubMed]
23. García-Gollarte, F.; Mora-Concepción, A.; Pinazo-Hernandis, S.; Segura-Ortí, E.; Amer-Cuenca, J.J.; Arguisuelas-Martínez, M.D.; Lisón, J.F.; Benavent-Caballer, V. Effectiveness of a Supervised Group-Based Otago Exercise Program on Functional Performance in Frail Institutionalized Older Adults: A Multicenter Randomized Controlled Trial. *J. Geriatr. Phys. Ther.* **2021**, in press. [CrossRef] [PubMed]
24. Ries, J.D.; Hutson, J.; Maralit, L.A.; Brown, M.B. Group Balance Training Specifically Designed for Individuals With Alzheimer Disease: Impact on Berg Balance Scale, Timed Up and Go, Gait Speed, and Mini-Mental Status Examination. *J. Geriatr. Phys. Ther.* **2015**, *38*, 183–193. [CrossRef] [PubMed]
25. Ries, J.D.; Drake, J.M.; Marino, C. A Small-Group Functional Balance Intervention for Individuals with Alzheimer Disease: A Pilot Study. *J. Neurol. Phys. Ther.* **2010**, *34*, 3–10. [CrossRef]
26. The Otago Exercise Program | Carolina Geriatric Workforce Enhancement Program (CGWEP). Available online: https://www.med.unc.edu/aging/cgwep/exercise-program/ (accessed on 2 February 2021).
27. Hoddinott, P. A New Era for Intervention Development Studies. *Pilot Feasibility Stud.* **2015**, *1*, 36. [CrossRef]
28. Folstein, M.F.M.; Folstein, S.E.S.; McHugh, P.R.P. "Mini-Mental State". A Practical Method for Grading the Cognitive State of Patients for the Clinician. *J. Psychiatr. Res.* **1975**, *12*, 189–198. [CrossRef]
29. Sclan, S.G.S.; Reisberg, B.B. Functional Assessment Staging (FAST) in Alzheimer's Disease: Reliability, Validity, and Ordinality. *Int. Psychogeriatr. IPA* **1992**, *4* (Suppl. 1), 55–69. [CrossRef]
30. Tombaugh, T.N.; McIntyre, N.J. The Mini-Mental State Examination: A Comprehensive Review. *J. Am. Geriatr. Soc.* **1992**, *40*, 922–935. [CrossRef]
31. STEADI-Older Adult Fall Prevention | CDC. Available online: https://www.cdc.gov/steadi/index.html (accessed on 31 January 2021).
32. Podsiadlo, D.D.; Richardson, S.S. The Timed "Up & Go": A Test of Basic Functional Mobility for Frail Elderly Persons. *J. Am. Geriatr. Soc.* **1991**, *39*, 142–148.
33. Ries, J.D.; Echternach, J.L.; Nof, L.; Blodgett, M.G. Test-Retest Reliability and Minimal Detectable Change Scores for the Timed "Up & Go" Test, the Six-Minute Walk Test, and Gait Speed in People With Alzheimer Disease. *Phys. Ther.* **2009**, *89*, 569–579.
34. National Center for Injury Prevention and Control, US DHHS. *Tools to Implement the Otago Exercise Program: A Program to Reduce Falls*, 1st ed.; National Center for Injury Prevention and Control: Atlanta, GA, USA, 2019. Available online: https://www.med.unc.edu/aging/cgwep/wp-content/uploads/sites/865/2018/09/ImplementationGuideforPT.pdf (accessed on 2 October 2021).
35. Lusardi, M.M.; Fritz, S.; Middleton, A.; Allison, L.; Wingood, M.; Phillips, E.; Criss, M.; Verma, S.; Osborne, J.; Chui, K.K. Determining Risk of Falls in Community Dwelling Older Adults: A Systematic Review and Meta-Analysis Using Posttest Probability. *J. Geriatr. Phys. Ther.* **2017**, *40*, 1–36. [CrossRef] [PubMed]
36. Jones, C.J.; Rikli, R.E.; Beam, W.C. A 30-s Chair-Stand Test as a Measure of Lower Body Strength in Community-Residing Older Adults. *Res. Q. Exerc. Sport* **1999**, *70*, 113–119. [CrossRef] [PubMed]
37. Hesseberg, K.; Bentzen, H.; Bergland, A. Reliability of the Senior Fitness Test in Community-Dwelling Older People with Cognitive Impairment. *Physiother. Res. Int. J. Res. Clin. Phys. Ther.* **2015**, *20*, 37–44. [CrossRef]
38. Rossiter-Fornoff, J.E.; Wolf, S.L.; Wolfson, L.I.; Buchner, D.M. A Cross-Sectional Validation Study of the FICSIT Common Data Base Static Balance Measures. Frailty and Injuries: Cooperative Studies of Intervention Techniques. *J. Gerontol. A Biol. Sci. Med. Sci.* **1995**, *50*, M291–M297. [CrossRef] [PubMed]
39. Bossers, W.J.R.; van der Woude, L.H.V.; Boersma, F.; Hortobágyi, T.; Scherder, E.J.A.; van Heuvelen, M.J.G. A 9-Week Aerobic and Strength Training Program Improves Cognitive and Motor Function in Patients with Dementia: A Randomized, Controlled Trial. *Am. J. Geriatr. Psychiatry* **2015**, *23*, 1106–1116. [CrossRef]
40. Blankevoort, C.G.; van Heuvelen, M.J.G.; Scherder, E.J.A. Reliability of Six Physical Performance Tests in Older People with Dementia. *Phys. Ther.* **2013**, *93*, 69–78. [CrossRef]
41. Murphy, M.A.; Olson, S.L.; Protas, E.J.; Overby, A.R. Screening for Falls in Community-Dwelling Elderly. *J. Aging Phys. Act.* **2003**, *11*, 66–80. [CrossRef]
42. Trautwein, S.; Maurus, P.; Barisch-Fritz, B.; Hadzic, A.; Woll, A. Recommended Motor Assessments Based on Psychometric Properties in Individuals with Dementia: A Systematic Review. *Eur. Rev. Aging Phys. Act.* **2019**, *16*, 20. [CrossRef]

43. McGough, E.L.; Lin, S.-Y.; Belza, B.; Becofsky, K.M.; Jones, D.L.; Liu, M.; Wilcox, S.; Logsdon, R.G. A Scoping Review of Physical Performance Outcome Measures Used in Exercise Interventions for Older Adults With Alzheimer Disease and Related Dementias. *J. Geriatr. Phys. Ther.* **2017**, *42*, 28–47. [CrossRef]
44. Ries, J.D. Rehabilitation for Individuals with Dementia: Facilitating Success. *Curr. Geriatr. Rep.* **2018**, *7*, 59–70. [CrossRef]
45. Conradsson, M.M.; Lundin-Olsson, L.L.; Lindelöf, N.N.; Littbrand, H.H.; Malmqvist, L.L.; Gustafson, Y.Y.; Rosendahl, E.E. Berg Balance Scale: Intrarater Test-Retest Reliability among Older People Dependent in Activities of Daily Living and Living in Residential Care Facilities. *Phys. Ther.* **2007**, *87*, 1155–1163. [CrossRef] [PubMed]
46. Kleim, J.A.; Jones, T.A. Principles of Experience-Dependent Neural Plasticity: Implications for Rehabilitation after Brain Damage. *J. Speech Lang. Hear. Res. JSLHR* **2008**, *51*, S225–S239. [CrossRef]
47. Di Lorito, C.; Bosco, A.; Booth, V.; Goldberg, S.; Harwood, R.H.; Van der Wardt, V. Adherence to Exercise Interventions in Older People with Mild Cognitive Impairment and Dementia: A Systematic Review and Meta-Analysis. *Prev. Med. Rep.* **2020**, *19*, 101139. [CrossRef] [PubMed]
48. Gonçalves, A.-C.; Cruz, J.; Marques, A.; Demain, S.; Samuel, D. Evaluating Physical Activity in Dementia: A Systematic Review of Outcomes to Inform the Development of a Core Outcome Set. *Age Ageing* **2018**, *47*, 34–41. [CrossRef] [PubMed]
49. McPhate, L.; Simek, E.M.; Haines, T.P.; Hill, K.D.; Finch, C.F.; Day, L. "Are Your Clients Having Fun?" The Implications of Respondents' Preferences for the Delivery of Group Exercise Programs for Falls Prevention. *J. Aging Phys. Act.* **2016**, *24*, 129–138. [CrossRef]
50. Booth, V.; Harwood, R.; Hancox, J.E.; Hood-Moore, V.; Masud, T.; Logan, P. Motivation as a Mechanism Underpinning Exercise-Based Falls Prevention Programmes for Older Adults with Cognitive Impairment: A Realist Review. *BMJ Open* **2019**, *9*, e024982. [CrossRef]
51. Lindelöf, N.; Lundin-Olsson, L.; Skelton, D.A.; Lundman, B.; Rosendahl, E. Experiences of Older People with Dementia Participating in a High-Intensity Functional Exercise Program in Nursing Homes: "While It's Tough, It's Useful". *PLoS ONE* **2017**, *12*, e0188225. [CrossRef]
52. Sherrington, C.; Whitney, J.C.; Lord, S.R.; Herbert, R.D.; Cumming, R.G.; Close, J.C.T. Effective Exercise for the Prevention of Falls: A Systematic Review and Meta-Analysis. *J. Am. Geriatr. Soc.* **2008**, *56*, 2234–2243. [CrossRef] [PubMed]
53. Meyer, C.; Hill, K.D.; Hill, S.; Dow, B. Falls Prevention for People with Dementia: A Knowledge Translation Intervention. *Dementia* **2019**, *19*, 2267–2293. [CrossRef]

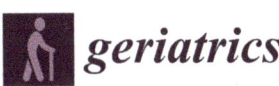

Case Report

Cognitive and Behavior Deficits in Parkinson's Disease with Alteration of FDG-PET Irrespective of Age

Fulvio Lauretani [1,2,*], Livia Ruffini [3], Crescenzo Testa [1], Marco Salvi [1], Mara Scarlattei [2], Giorgio Baldari [2], Irene Zucchini [1], Beatrice Lorenzi [1], Chiara Cattabiani [1] and Marcello Maggio [1]

[1] Department of Medicine and Surgery, University of Parma, 43124 Parma, Italy; crescenzo.testa@unipr.it (C.T.); marco.salvi@unipr.it (M.S.); irene.zucchini@unipr.it (I.Z.); beatrice.lorenzi@unipr.it (B.L.); chiarac2004@libero.it (C.C.); marcellogiuseppe.maggio@unipr.it (M.M.)
[2] Geriatric Clinic, Geriatric-Rehabilitation Department, University Hospital, 43124 Parma, Italy; mscarlattei@ao.pr.it (M.S.); gbaldari@ao.pr.it (G.B.)
[3] Nuclear Medicine Division, University-Hospital of Parma, 43124 Parma, Italy; lruffini@ao.pr.it
* Correspondence: fulvio.lauretani@unipr.it

Abstract: Significant progress has been made in our understanding of the neurobiology of Parkinson's disease (PD). Post-mortem studies are an important step and could help to comprehend not only the progression of motor symptoms, but also the involvement of other clinical domains, including cognition, behavior and impulse control disorders (ICDs). The correlation of neuropathological extension of the disease with the clinical stages remains challenging. Molecular imaging, including positron emission tomography (PET) and single photon computed tomography (SPECT), could allow for bridging the gap by providing in vivo evidence of disease extension. In the last decade, we have observed a plethora of reports describing improvements in the sensitivity of neuroimaging techniques. These data contribute to increasing the accuracy of PD diagnosis, differentiating PD from other causes of parkinsonism and also obtaining a surrogate marker of disease progression. FDG-PET has been used to measure cerebral metabolic rates of glucose, a proxy for neuronal activity, in PD. Many studies have shown that this technique could be used in early PD, where reduced metabolic activity correlates with disease progression and could predict histopathological diagnosis. The aim of this work is to report two particular cases of PD in which the assessment of brain metabolic activity (from FDG-PET) has been combined with clinical aspects of non-motor symptoms. Integration of information on neuropsychological and metabolic imaging allows us to improve the treatment of PD patients irrespective of age.

Keywords: molecular imaging; ICDs; 18F-FDG-PET; Parkinson's disease; dopamine agonists

1. Introduction

Parkinson's disease (PD) is an age-related neurodegenerative disorder that affects as many as 1–2% of people aged 60 years and older [1]. The incidence and prevalence of this disease are constantly growing, mainly due to the aging of the population [2]. It has been estimated that the annual incidence ranges from 5/100.000 to over 35/100.000 new cases, with a 5–10-fold increase from the sixth to the ninth decade of life [3,4]. The prevalence of the disease also increases with age. In a meta-analysis of four North American populations, the prevalence of the disease was shown to increase from nearly 1% in the first 55 years of life to over 4% in men over 85 years of age.

Lower prevalence values were found in women with "only" 2% of women affected by the disease when over 85 years of age [5]. Despite the serious impact on the quality of life of patients, which can be mitigated by the treatments that will be discussed later, the mortality in these patients is equal to those unaffected by PD in the first ten years from diagnosis, and tends to increase later [6].

It is evident that in older populations, which are more predisposed to developing neurodegenerative diseases such as Parkinson's disease, the social and economic aspects deriving from this epidemiological framework will be increasingly important [7,8]. Therefore, in the therapeutic approach of this disease, it is fundamental to avoid treatments that can contribute themselves to lowering the quality of life, not only of patients, but also of caregivers who are central figures in the standards of care of this disease [9].

Impulse control disorders are one of the side effects that most negatively impact the quality of life of patients and their caregivers under dopamine replacement therapies. Other disorders including pathological gambling, compulsive sexual behavior and buying, and binge or compulsive eating have been described [10]. These disorders generally affect younger patients and those who have first-degree relatives in the family in whom similar problems have been described, regardless of the diagnosis of Parkinson's disease [11]. Although ICDs have been associated with high dose levodopa treatment, it is important to note that this side effect is significantly more pronounced in patients receiving dopamine agonists [11]. The reason for this association is unclear, but one of the most probable hypotheses is based on the affinity profile of dopaminergic agonists for some dopamine receptor isoforms. In fact, while the motor effects of dopamine replacement therapies are due to dopamine D1 and D2 receptors, ICDs are due to an effect on dopamine D3 receptors [12]. D3 receptors are mostly expressed in the ventral striatum [12], a prosencephalic region associated with both behavioral addictions [13] and substance abuse disorders [14].

It has been shown that especially new dopaminergic agonists (ropinirole and pramipexole) have greater selectivity for D3 receptors than for D1 and D2 dopamine receptors [15]. It is therefore evident that we are no longer faced, as has been hypothesized for a long time, with a disease with only implications on motor functions. In 2003, Braak and colleagues already hypothesized a neuroanatomic staging of the disease affecting different domains (Braak's stages 1 and 2 are associated with the premotor phase; Braak's stages 3–4 are associated with the motor symptoms; and Braak's stages 5–6 are associated with cognitive impairment) [16].

Taking into account the complexity of symptomatology of PD, it becomes important to plan an appropriate treatment to balance motor and cognitive and behavior symptoms of the patient [17].

In fact, L-dopa or dopamine agonists may produce neuropsychiatric side effects not only in relation of the age of the patient but also if the patient presents some degree of cognitive impairment or psychiatric symptoms such as ICDs.

PET with 18F-fluorodeoxyglucose (FDG-PET) has been used to measure regional cerebral glucose metabolism, a proxy for neuronal activity, in PD. Many studies have shown that this technique could be used in early PD, where reduced metabolic activity correlates with disease progression and predict histopathological diagnosis [18].

The clinical usefulness of introducing PET-FDG in the therapeutic work-up of Parkinson's disease is not only related to the increase in sensitivity and diagnostic specificity, but also in improving the stratification of patients, thus increasingly promoting personalized medicine.

First of all, the PET-FDG describes hypometabolism patterns typical of Parkinson's disease (Parkinson's Disease Related Pattern, PDRP) [17]. Furthermore, unlike other techniques, PET-FDG offers high sensitivity with admirable spatial and temporal resolution. It is also important to underline that unlike the DAT-scan, PET-FDG is able to highlight hypometabolisms not only in the dopaminergic pathways, but also in other receptor pathways upstream or downstream of these. In this way, while keeping in mind the fundamental importance of dopaminergic pathways in the pathogenesis of Parkinson's disease, it is also possible to investigate other receptor pathways certainly involved in the development of non-motor disorders [19].

The aim of this work is to report on particular cases of PD in which assessment of cerebral metabolic activity (from FDG-PET) has been combined with clinical evaluation of non-motor symptoms. Integration of clinical and metabolic imaging information provide to better treat patients with PD irrespective of age.

2. Methods

Patients were evaluated at the Cognitive and Motor Ambulatory of the Geriatric-Rehabilitation Department of the University Hospital of Parma, while the FDG-PET scans were performed at the Nuclear Medicine Department of University Hospital of Parma (Parma, Italy). Patients were first evaluated by an expert geriatrician with a standard clinical evaluation [20,21] and then referred to a psychologist with long-term experience in the evaluation of older persons because of complaints of neuro-psychiatric symptoms. Diagnosis of PD was made according to Movement Disorders Society (MDS) criteria [22], while all cognitive tests included in the neuropsychology battery have norms and cut-offs available for the Italian population [21]. The 15 item Geriatric Depression Scale (GDS) was used for assessing depression [23] and the Wisconsin Card Sorting Test was used to examine aspects of executive function [21]. All patients had a recent MRI or CT scan. All drug consumption was recorded. The two patients gave the consent to record these data. They are enrolled in the prospective observational T.R.I.P. Study (Traumatic Risk Identikit Parma Study). (The study was approved by the Ethical Committee of the University Hospital of Parma, ID 17262 del 12/05/2017). Data were treated in agreement with Italian law for the privacy guaranty.

2.1. 18F-FDG PET/CT

An 18F-FDG scan was performed using a whole-body hybrid system Discovery IQ (GE Healthcare) operating in three-dimensional detection mode. A head holder was used to restrict patient movement and head movement was checked on a regular basis.

After an overnight fast, 200 MBq of 18F-FDG was administered intravenously in a quiet, dimly lit examination room. The brain PET/CT recording was started 30 min after tracer injection. During the 30-min uptake period, participants were left undisturbed in a darkened room and instructed to rest quietly without activity with their eyes closed, as is commonly recommended. The brain CT was first recorded to provide the attenuation correction map (140 kV, 25 mA, 512 × 512 matrix, 3.75-mm slice thickness, scan Type Helical full 0.8 s, No of images 79, Rec Fov 30 cm, recon type standard). CT was immediately followed by a 3D-PET recording during a 10-min period (FOV 30 cm, recon type QCHD and VPHD, matrix size 256 × 256). Quantitative analysis was performed using the SPM5 software implemented in Matlab R2014a [24].

The patient PET dataset is spatially normalized using the SPM5 PET template and smoothed with a Gaussian filter of 8 mm FWHM. Differences in CMRglc (patient vs. normal) are assessed on a voxel-by-voxel basis, using a paired t-test. The results are displayed on the Tailarach atlas.

2.2. Example of Young and Older PD Patient Showing ICDs after Using Dopamine Agonists: Evaluation with FDG-PET

2.2.1. First Case (Young Patient: PD with ICDs after Using Ropinirole)

A 55-year-old man with resting tremor and rigidity was evaluated at the Cognitive and Motor Ambulatory, University Hospital of Parma. His medical history was characterized by presence of diabetes, hypertension and chronic ischemic coronaropathy. At the first visit a resting tremor at the right hand and plastic rigidity with "lead-pipe" rigidity was observed. Given the multimorbidity of the patients, a SPECT with 123I-ioflupane (DaTSCAN©) (Figure 1) was prescribed. The exam showed reduced uptake in dopamine making the diagnosis of PD probable, according to the MDS criteria. Mini Mental Examination State (MMSE) score was normal (30/30 corrected for age and education) as well as cerebral MRI. Initially, a standard dose of dopamine agonists, ropinirole extended release was prescribed, and even if motor symptoms one year later were reduced, the patient's wife reported a strange behavior, including excess of shopping and changes of sexuality with clear hypersexuality.

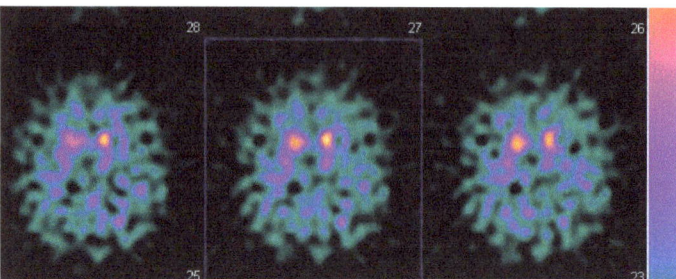

Figure 1. Brain SPECT with 123 I-iofuplain (DaTSCAN).

Given psychiatric symptoms reported, we changed the current treatment starting L-dopa and prescribed the FDG-PET, because of the severe anxiety induced in family members of this young PD patient. FDG-PET showed extended hypometabolism in the right and left inferior frontal gyrus and in part of the prefrontal lateral areas (Figure 2). A further cognitive assessment by MMSE remained normal and even the second level of neuropsychological evaluation resulted normal. After the prescription of L-dopa at the dosage of 300 mg daily, motor symptoms disappeared and patient's wife reported a profound improvement of behavior, with disappearance of ICDs.

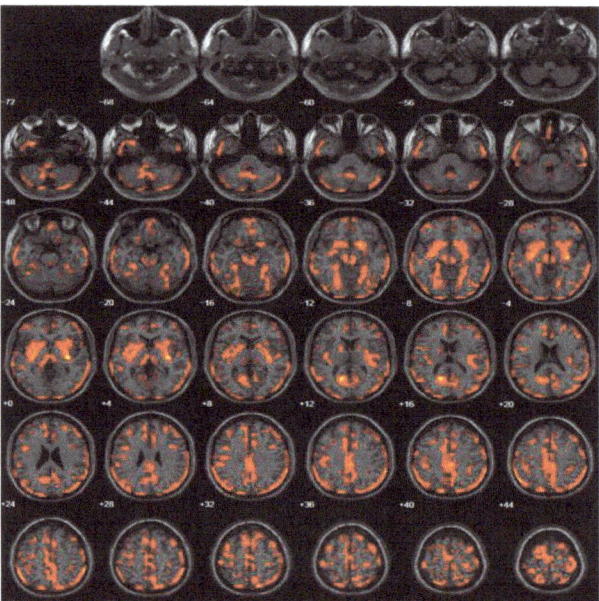

Figure 2. Brain PET with 18F-FDG. Images highlight brain regions consistently found the analysis (Statistical Parametric Mapping software SPM 5 ($p = 0.05$). Diffuse hypometabolism in the left middle temporal gyrus, right and left inferior frontal gyrus, left middle frontal gyrus, left posterior cingulate, left inferior parietal lobule, right lentiform nucleus (putamen), right caudate head, left thalamus, left parahippocampal gyrus, right red nucleus (midbrain), left cerebellum pyramis, right and left cerebellum inferior semi-lunar lobule, right and left cerebellum posterior lobe tuber, right cerebellum anterior lobe nodule, left cerebellar tonsil.

2.2.2. Second Case (Older Patient: PD with ICDs after Using Pramipexole)

A 70-year-old man with established diagnosis of PD suggested by a private neurologist, was evaluated at the Cognitive and Motor Ambulatory, University Hospital of Parma, two years after the diagnosis. All cardinal motor symptoms were present, with an evident association of depression as non-motor symptom. The patient used pramipexole as first drug prescribed by neurologist, but he reported a motoric difficult to perform activities of daily living. Thus, he asked us to revise dosage or change the drug. He was retired from his principal work, but he was still involved as a lecturer in theology. At the initial cognitive assessment, he showed a normal MMSE (30/30 corrected for age and education). The evaluation included a structured neurological visit without evidence of neurological clinical signs. The patient's wife reported an increase of sexuality, completely unexpected in relation to the past behavior and given his catholic principles. The patient received the second-stage cognitive screening by an expert psychologist and logopedist and the evaluation resulted normal.

Given the reported ICDs, we changed treatment using L-dopa and prescribed the FDG-PET, to exclude other forms of parkinsonism. The FDG-PET scan showed hypometabolism in many cerebral areas involving, also in this case, the right and left inferior frontal gyrus and part of the prefrontal lateral areas (Figure 3). After the prescription of L-dopa at the dosage of 400 mg daily, we also added venlafaxine for improving depressive symptoms. After a 5-year follow-up period, the patient reported a discrete control of motor symptoms, e.g., he drove his car for more than two hours, and his wife reported a completely disappearance of ICDs, with significant improvement of behavior returning to the same as before starting treatment.

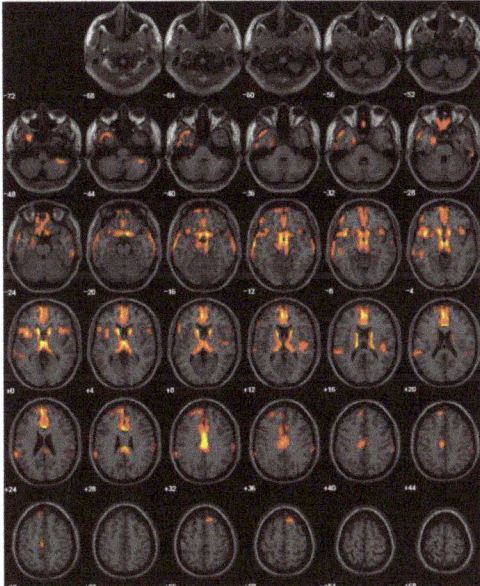

Figure 3. Brain PET with 18F-FDG. Images highlight brain regions consistently found the analysis (Statistical Parametric Mapping software SPM 5 ($p = 0.05$). Hypometabolism in the left caudate body and head, left middle temporal gyrus, left superior temporal gyrus, right superior frontal gyrus, left and right inferior parietal lobule, left and right cerebrum sub-lobar insula, left and right superior temporal gyrus, left and right inferior frontal gyrus, right sub-lobar extra-nuclear gray matter, right cerebellar tonsil, right inferior temporal gyrus, left and right middle temporal gyrus, left limbic lobe uncus, left limbic lobe parahippocampal gyrus, right transverse temporal gyrus.

3. Discussion on the Integration of Neuropsychological and Neuroimaging Information

The dopaminergic system is mainly composed in two ways: 1. the Nigro-Striatal system, rich in D1 and D2 dopaminergic receptors, which are responsible of the movement; and 2. Meso-Limbic and prefrontal cortex-ventral striatal systems, where are mainly found D3 and D4 dopaminergic receptors, which are responsible for the positive symptoms of schizophrenia such as hallucinations and delusions. Direct consequences of alteration of these pathways, and in particular of the "prefrontal cortex-ventral striatal systems", when using dopamine agonists, could be the developing of ICDs even in an initial phase of the disease. Previously, we have shown that dopamine agonists have a greater selectivity for D3 receptors [15]. A recent study showed that treatment with dopamine agonists interferes with the functional activity of the prefrontal cortex and the ventral striatum [25]. Regardless of dopamine agonist treatment, in patients who had a greater tendency to develop ICDs there was less functional activity in the right inferior frontal gyrus [25]. The importance of the inferior frontal gyrus in the inhibition of impulsive controls was already described in the literature. The presence of lesions in this region, regardless of Parkinson's disease, can cause ICDs [26].

All these data support what was reported by Ruppert MC and colleagues, who showed that high impulsivity, defined as a personality trait, predisposes to risk-seeking behavior, and is closely associated with impaired FDG-metabolism within the fronto-insula network in PD [27].

ICDs seem to be caused by a heterogeneous melting pot of predisposing factors independent of Parkinson's disease together with an altered response to dopamine agonist therapies.

The development of an ICD can be compared with an "epileptic seizure" where different triggers (dopamine agonist treatment) work above an epileptogenic substrate (personal trait of developing ICD, in particular a reduced activity in the inferior frontal gyrus). In this direction, the utilization of FDG-PET to detect a metabolic alteration in the inferior frontal gyrus could orient clinician's in selecting the most appropriate drug for PD treatment.

Over the years, an increasing number of physicians started to use dopamine agonists in younger patients confining levodopa treatment to the most advanced stages of the disease [28].

However, early levodopa treatment, in addition to be effective at all patient's age, does not interfere with the progression of the disease [29,30]. Although dopamine agonists predispose to side effects such as ICDs [31], their use remains fundamental given the well-known and greater risk of developing dyskinesias induced by levodopa.

Correct stratification of patients in the initial stages of the disease is therefore essential to decide the most appropriate treatment. The presented case reports permit to support the use of molecular imaging with FDG-PET for selecting drugs in the early phase of PD, even in patients with a medical history negative for significant psychiatric symptoms.

The limitations of our study may be to suggest a PET scan with relatively high costs, when the full clinical evaluation could be realized with an exhaustive explanation of the side-effects of dopamine agonists. However, FDG-PET could reinforce reasons why these medications produce ICDs only in some patients. Furthermore, our report is based on data from only two patients. It would be improper to generalize our conclusions to the general population: for this reason, further studies are needed to investigate whether our conclusions can be generalized to the general population. It would be important, in the diagnostic/therapeutic flow-chart of Parkinson's disease, a method that not only increases the sensitivity and specificity in making the diagnosis, but that stratifies patients in order to propose a treatment as personalized as possible, so as to propose an increasingly personalized medicine. From this perspective, the cost effectiveness of proposing a diagnostic investigation that still remains expensive would also improve.

Many therapeutic options have become available for PD in recent years, leading to significant improvements in motor control both at early and advanced disease stages [31]. The need to expand disease management beyond motor symptoms control has been recently highlighted [32]. There is recent evidence that on-motor features deeply affect the quality of life of patients [33].

Dopamine agonists represent a valid therapeutic option in PD and their effects on non-motor domains like mood or cognition are acknowledged as key factors in fully addressing patients' needs.

The balance between motor deficits and cognitive or psychiatric symptoms seems to be the most important factor contributing to treatment decision-making when approaching PD therapy.

In conclusion, earlier [17] and more accurate diagnosis of PD with impaired all dopaminergic pathways may help to improve patient's health status and reduce treatment costs by effectively allocating healthcare resources and maximizing the benefit of treatments and supportive services.

Use of FDG-PET may help to accurately identify PD patients that could develop ICDs after using dopamine agonists.

Unlike previous works [19], our approach is not so much aimed at demonstrating the diagnostic utility of PET-FDG in Parkinson's disease, but is aimed, instead, at a better stratification of patients so as to prevent serious side effects that, in predisposed patients, can lead to serious consequences. Furthermore, with PET-FDG it is possible to discriminate certain hypometabolism patterns significant for cognitive deterioration. Recent evidence indicates that these patients are also more predisposed to the development of ICDs [34].

The development of novel model of clusters of PD patients [35] may provide additional benefits by slowing or halting progressive decline of PD, increasing quality of life and prolonging survival.

Funding: This research received no external funding.

Institutional Review Board Statement: The study was approved by the Ethical Committee of the University Hospital of Parma, ID 17262 del 12/05/2017.

Informed Consent Statement: Informed consent was obtained from all subjects involved in the study.

Data Availability Statement: Not applicable.

Acknowledgments: The authors do not have any conflict of interest in the publication of this case report, have all contributed to the conception of the description and in the writing of this case report, and have approved the manuscript in its present form.

Conflicts of Interest: The authors declare no conflict of interest.

References

1. Zhang, S.; Smailagic, N. (11)C-PIB-PET for the early diagnosis of Alzheimer's disease dementia and other dementias in people with mild cognitive impairment (MCI). *Cochrane Database Syst. Rev.* **2014**, *7*. [CrossRef] [PubMed]
2. Hou, Y.; Dan, X. Ageing as a risk factor for neurodegenerative disease. *Nat. Rev. Neurol.* **2019**, *15*, 565–581. [CrossRef] [PubMed]
3. Twelves, D.; Perkins, K.S. Systematic review of incidence studies of Parkinson's disease. *Mov. Disord.* **2003**, *18*, 19–31. [CrossRef] [PubMed]
4. Poewe, W.; Seppi, K. Parkinson disease. *Nat. Rev. Dis. Primers* **2017**, *3*, 17013. [CrossRef]
5. Marras, C.; Beck, J.C. Parkinson's Foundation P4 Group. Prevalence of Parkinson's disease across North America. *NPJ Parkinsons Dis.* **2018**, *4*, 21. [CrossRef]
6. Pinter, B.; Diem-Zangerl, A. Mortality in Parkinson's disease: A 38-year follow-up study. *Mov. Disord.* **2015**, *30*, 266–269. [CrossRef]
7. Dorsey, E.R.; Sherer, T. The Emerging Evidence of the Parkinson Pandemic. *J. Parkinsons Dis.* **2018**, *8*, S3–S8. [CrossRef]
8. Kaltenboeck, A.; Johnson, S.J. Direct costs and survival of medicare beneficiaries with early and advanced Parkinson's disease. *Parkinsonism Relat. Disord.* **2012**, *18*, 321–326. [CrossRef] [PubMed]
9. Mosley, P.E.; Moodie, R. Caregiver Burden in Parkinson Disease: A Critical Review of Recent Literature. *J. Geriatr. Psychiatry Neurol.* **2017**, *30*, 235–252. [CrossRef]
10. Voon, V.; Fox, S.H. Medication-related impulse control and repetitive behaviors in Parkinson disease. *Arch. Neurol.* **2007**, *64*, 1089–1096. [CrossRef]
11. Weintraub, D.; Koester, J. Impulse control disorders in Parkinson disease: A cross-sectional study of 3090 patients. *Arch. Neurol.* **2010**, *67*, 589–595. [CrossRef]

12. Gurevich, E.V.; Joyce, J.N. Distribution of dopamine D3 receptor expressing neurons in the human forebrain: Comparison with D2 receptor expressing neurons. *Neuropsychopharmacology* **1999**, *20*, 60–80. [CrossRef]
13. Holden, C. 'Behavioral' addictions: Do they exist? *Science* **2001**, *294*, 980–982. [CrossRef] [PubMed]
14. Brewer, J.A.; Potenza, M.N. The neurobiology and genetics of impulse control disorders: Relationships to drug addictions. *Biochem. Pharmacol.* **2008**, *75*, 63–75. [CrossRef] [PubMed]
15. Gerlach, M.; Double, K. Dopamine receptor agonists in current clinical use: Comparative dopamine receptor binding profiles defined in the human striatum. *J. Neural. Transm.* **2003**, *110*, 1119–1127. [CrossRef]
16. Braak, H.; Del Tredici, K. Staging of brain pathology related to sporadic Parkinson's disease. *Neurobiol. Aging* **2003**, *24*, 197–211. [CrossRef]
17. Armstrong, M.J.; Okun, M.S. Diagnosis and Treatment of Parkinson Disease: A Review. *JAMA* **2020**, *323*, 548–560. [CrossRef] [PubMed]
18. Matthews, D.C.; Lerman, H. FDG PET Parkinson's disease-related pattern as a biomarker for clinical trials in early stage disease. *Neuroimage Clin.* **2018**, *20*, 572–579. [CrossRef]
19. Walker, Z.; Gandolfo, F. Clinical utility of FDG PET in Parkinson's disease and atypical parkinsonism associated with dementia. *Eur. J. Nucl. Med. Mol. Imaging* **2018**, *45*, 1534–1545. [CrossRef] [PubMed]
20. Ferrucci, L.; Bandinelli, S. Neurological examination findings to predict limitations in mobility and falls in older persons without a history of neurological disease. *Am. J. Med.* **2004**, *116*, 807–815. [CrossRef]
21. Caffarra, P.; Ghetti, C. Differential patterns of hypoperfusion in subtypes of mild cognitive impairment. *Open Neuroimag. J.* **2008**, *2*, 20–28. [CrossRef] [PubMed]
22. Postuma, R.B.; Berg, D. MDS clinical diagnostic criteria for Parkinson's disease. *Mov. Disord.* **2015**, *30*, 1591–1601. [CrossRef] [PubMed]
23. Yesavage, J.A.; Brink, T.L. Development and validation of a geriatric depression screening scale: A preliminary report. *J. Psychiatr. Res.* **1982–1983**, *17*, 37–49. [CrossRef]
24. Good, C.D.; Johnsrude, I.S. A voxel-based morphometric study of ageing in 465 normal adult human brains. *Neuroimage* **2001**, *14 Pt 1*, 21–36. [CrossRef] [PubMed]
25. Haagensen, B.N.; Herz, D.M. Linking brain activity during sequential gambling to impulse control in Parkinson's disease. *Neuroimage Clin.* **2020**, *27*, 102330. [CrossRef]
26. Aron, A.R.; Robbins, T.W. Inhibition and the right inferior frontal cortex. *Trends Cogn. Sci.* **2004**, *8*, 170–177. [CrossRef]
27. Ruppert, M.C.; Greuel, A. Network degeneration in Parkinson's disease: Multimodal imaging of nigro-striato-cortical dysfunction. *Brain* **2020**, *143*, 944–959. [CrossRef]
28. Connolly, B.S.; Lang, A.E. Pharmacological treatment of Parkinson disease: A review. *JAMA* **2014**, *311*, 1670–1683. [CrossRef] [PubMed]
29. Espay, A.J.; Lang, A.E. Common Myths in the Use of Levodopa in Parkinson Disease: When Clinical Trials Misinform Clinical Practice. *JAMA Neurol.* **2017**, *74*, 633–634. [CrossRef]
30. Gray, R.; Ives, N. Long-term effectiveness of dopamine agonists and monoamine oxidase B inhibitors compared with levodopa as initial treatment for Parkinson's disease (PD MED): A large, open-label, pragmatic randomised trial. *Lancet* **2014**, *384*, 1196–1205.
31. Garcia-Ruiz, P.J.; Martinez Castrillo, J.C. Impulse control disorder in patients with Parkinson's disease under dopamine agonist therapy: A multicentre study. *J. Neurol. Neurosurg. Psychiatry* **2014**, *85*, 840–844. [CrossRef] [PubMed]
32. Eidelberg, D.; Moeller, J.R. The metabolic topography of parkinsonism. *J. Cereb. Blood Flow Metab.* **1994**, *14*, 783–801. [CrossRef] [PubMed]
33. Chang, A.; Fox, S.H. Psychosis in Parkinson's Disease: Epidemiology, Pathophysiology, and Management. *Drugs* **2016**, *76*, 1093–1118. [CrossRef] [PubMed]
34. Martinez-Martin, P.; Wan, Y.M. Impulse control and related behaviors in Parkinson's disease with dementia. *Eur. J. Neurol.* **2020**, *27*, 944–950. [CrossRef] [PubMed]
35. Lauretani, F.; Longobucco, Y. Imaging the Functional Neuroanatomy of Parkinson's Disease: Clinical Applications and Future Directions. *Int. J. Environ. Res. Public Health* **2021**, *18*, 2356. [CrossRef] [PubMed]

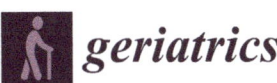

Case Report

A Case Study on Polypharmacy and Depression in a 75-Year-Old Woman with Visual Deficits and Charles Bonnet Syndrome

José Caamaño-Ponte [1], Martina Gómez Digón [2], Mercedes Pereira Pía [3], Antonio de la Iglesia Cabezudo [3], Margarita Echevarría Canoura [4] and David Facal [5,*]

1. Grupo de Investigación Dependencia, Gerontología, y Geriatría, Universidade Santiago de Compostela, 15782 Santiago de Compostela, Spain; caamajos@hotmail.com
2. Servicio Enfermería EOXI Lugo, 27003 Lugo, Spain; marttina24@gmail.com
3. Servicio Farmacia EOXI Lugo, 27003 Lugo, Spain; Maria.Mercedes.Pereira.Pia@sergas.es (M.P.P.); antonioluis.de.la.iglesia.cabezudo@sergas.es (A.d.l.I.C.)
4. Sanitas Hospitales A Coruña, 15005 A Coruna, Spain; mechevarriac@sanitas.es
5. Departamento de Psicología Evolutiva y de la Educación, Universidade de Santiago de Compostela, 15782 Santiago de Compostela, Spain
* Correspondence: david.facal@usc.es

Abstract: Depression is one of the most prevalent pathologies in older adults. Its diagnosis and treatment are complex due to different factors that intervene in its development and progression, including intercurrent organic diseases, perceptual deficits, use of drugs, and psycho-social conditions associated with the aging process. We present the case of a 75-year-old woman (who lives in the community) with a diagnosis of major depression with more than 10 years of history, analyzing her evolution and therapeutic approach.

Keywords: depression; adjustment disorder; glaucoma; hallucinations; polypharmacy

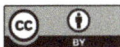

1. Introduction

Depressive disorders are the most common psychiatric pathology in old adulthood. It is associated with various mental and biological stressors that affect the functional capacity and independence of old adults, reducing their quality of life. International studies show variable prevalences that range between 8.8% and 23.6% in Europe [1,2], could reach 60% in Latin America, and would exceed 38% in rural Asian populations. This geographical variability is due to methodological, clinical, and sociocultural differences. Recent studies in Spain inform that up to 36% of older people living in urban areas in the community suffer from depression [3–5]. Depression seems to be more frequent in the female sex. However, this observation could be biased because women present a greater longevity and/or a greater tendency to go to medical services than men, whereas men present a more severe somatic expression of psychiatric symptoms and/or a higher reluctance to express psychiatric symptoms than women [6].

Depressive symptoms include affective disorders such as sadness, apathy, emotional lability and crying, anhedonia, and nihilism; behavior modifications such as anxiety, irritability, insomnia, and hyporexia; and alterations in the course and content of thought, as well as cognitive and physical frailty. Among all the symptoms, autolytic ideation requires a specific comment, since depression is the main suicide risk factor in old age. Suicide constitutes one of the 10 main causes of death in the old adults, mainly in men aged 65 and over who use more lethal methods conditioned by loneliness and isolation [7,8]. In old populations, the etiology of depression is multifactorial: there are psychosocial causes derived from the aging process (family losses, work life, loneliness, environmental barriers, lack of resources, lack of social support) in addition to genetic and biological factors that contribute to the increase in frailty, geriatric syndromes, and dependency [9,10].

Its diagnosis is clinical, following the criteria included in the International Classification of Diseases (ICD-10) or the Diagnostic and Statistical Manual of Mental Disorders (DSM-5, APA 2014). In old adults, the diagnosis can be complex due to comorbidity and drugs that potentially induce psychiatric symptoms and iatrogenic complications, to adaptive disorders following age-related changes and/or to incipient cognitive impairments. In any case, it can be an underdiagnosed disease due to circumstances related to its own nature, personality factors, and, also, because of the peculiarities of the healthcare systems [11].

To optimize its treatment, a transdisciplinary approach is required based on antidepressant drugs, such as selective serotonin reuptake inhibitors (SSRIs) or serotonin and norepinephrine reuptake inhibitors (SSNRIs), which have shown different therapeutic efficacy. It may also require, in many cases, mood stabilizers, anxiolytics, antipsychotics, tricyclic antidepressants (TCAs), or monoamine oxidase inhibitors (MAOIs) [12–14], plus psychosocial approaches (cognitive-behavioral psychotherapy, supportive psychotherapy), occupational techniques (re-education in activities of daily living, training in the use of technical aids), and physical training, which help to improve the prognosis and prevent relapses [15].

Within the different age-related conditions that can interfere with the diagnosis of depression in old age, Charles Bonnet syndrome is characterized by the presence of complex visual hallucinations, triggered by vision deprivation in the absence of neurological, psychiatric, and/or systemic disorders. The patient usually perceives the hallucinations as not real, which reduces anxiety, although the content, duration, and frequency are variable. Charles Bonnet syndrome can be associated with age-related entities such as enucleation, optic neuritis, diabetic retinopathy, macular degeneration, cataracts, and glaucoma, among others. Accordingly, its prevalence is relatively high in geriatric patients. In patients with major depression, a differential diagnosis with psychotic disorders is required [16,17].

The main objective of the study has been to facilitate deliberation on the frequent interrelation between organic pathologies, depressive symptomatology, and their overlap in time in old patients, as well as to present the heterodox therapeutic approach in this case, taking into account the complexity of the health care model of the Autonomous Community of Galicia (northwest Spain) and the patient's therapeutic choices.

2. Case

2.1. Personal History

A 75-year-old woman, who is right-handed, and a resident of the urban area of the province of A Coruña (Galicia, NW of Spain). She is married and has two children (one female and one male) and two male grandchildren. She lives with her husband (74 years old), who provides care support for the patient's visual deficits. A medium education of schooling is possessed, along with an administrative profession and adequate social resources.

2.2. Ethical Standards

The study was conducted in accordance with the "Request for authorization for access and publication of health data as clinical case/case series" as provided in the General Data Protection Regulation (EU Regulation 2016/679 of the European Parliament and of the Council, 27 April 2016) and the Spanish regulations on personal data protection in force. Written informed consent was obtained from the participant. Due to visual deficits in the patient, the informed consent was read aloud and supervised by the caregiver.

2.3. Medical History

According to medical records, during this study the patient presented hypothyroidism, dyslipidemia, type II diabetes mellitus, macular degeneration, glaucoma, arterial hypertension, hypertensive heart disease, ChadsVasc4 persistent atrial fibrillation, extensive calcification of the mitral annulus, mild mitral regurgitation, moderate tricuspid regurgitation, lacunar stroke, vertigo, peripheral vascular disease, bronchial asthma, and acute bronchitis progressively diagnosed. The patient demonstrates no toxic habits.

The patient has been followed by the family medicine (FM) service of the center since the end of 2013, with the aim of carrying out a preventive approach, in coordination with doctors from other specialties such as cardiology, endocrinology, ophthalmology, neurology, and psychiatry.

In the initial clinical evaluation, previously diagnosed diseases were treated with levothyroxine sodium, Armolipid Plus, a nutraceutical based on berberine, red yeast, policosanols, coenzyme Q10, astaxanthin and folic acid, and Bimatoprost solution, to which clonazepam and duloxetine were added to treat anxiety-depression symptoms. The general physical examination showed no data of interest. A control analysis was requested, whose most significant results were glucose in serum/plasma 156 mg/dL, total cholesterol 300 mg/dL, HDL 48 mg/dL, LDL 232 mg/dL, TSH 0.93 mIU/L, and the need was emphasized for diet and physical exercise to adjust lipid levels, explaining that the patient ruled out lipid-lowering drug treatment due to fear of liver damage. The FM insisted on the convenience of carrying out a scheduled follow-up.

Between 2014 and 2018, the patient went to her FM and specialist doctors on different occasions to control her chronic diseases (mainly hypothyroidism, dyslipidaemia, Diabetes Mellitus, and Glaucoma). Acute diseases such as respiratory infection, viriasis, oral candidiasis, lump infectious breast, sciatica, or sacral-coccygeal trauma were successfully treated. She also received systematic immunization against the influenza virus. She underwent surgery for her visual pathology in 2016, with relative success and maintenance treatment consisting of Lutein, Bimatoprost, and Brinzolamide. Bronchial asthma with treated with Budesonide/Formoterol. Table 1 shows the main pharmacological treatment modifications made to date.

Table 1. Evolutive drug adjustments.

Drugs/Year	2014	2018	2019	2020	2021-1	2021-2
Levotiroxina	100	100	100	100	100	100
Metformina	-	-	850	850	1275	1275
Espironolactona	25	25	25	-	-	-
Digoxina	-	-	125	125	125	125
Diltiazem R	-	-	120	120	120	120
Azetazolamida	-	-	250	250	250	250
Boi-K	-	-	1 c	1 c	1 c	1 c
Edobaxan	-	-	60	60	60	60
Armolipid/Lipok	'1 c	1 c	1 c	1 c	1 c	1 c
Ezetimiba	-	10	10	10	10	10
Atorvastatina	-	10	-	-	-	-
Duloxetina	60	60	-	-	-	-
Citalopram	-	-	10	-	-	-
Venlafaxin R	-	-	-	150	150	150
Venlafaxin	-	-	-	75	75	75
Mirtazapine	-	-	-	-	15	15
Lorazepam	1	1	1	1	1	1
Clonazepam	0.6	0.6	0.6	-	-	0.6

Note: 2021-1 (February 2021). 2021-2 (October 2021). Boi-K: Potassium hydrogen carbonate 1001 mg and ascorbic acid 250 mg, with dose in mgs. c: capsule.

2.4. History of the Disease

The prevalent symptomatology referred to by the patient and her family throughout the depressive process consists of sadness, emotional lability and crying, low self-esteem, negativism, apathy, anxiety, insomnia, ruminant thinking, and occasional autolytic ideation. Regarding the loss of visual capacity and the secondary dependence to it, the diagnosis of glaucoma and macular degeneration has been subsequent to the onset of depressive symptoms.

Over the years, an evolution characterized by periods of emotional well-being with a significant reduction in symptoms and different relapses that required therapeutic adjustments has been observed. Monitoring of the depressive disorder is carried out by a psychiatrist outside the primary care center, who adjusts the psychotropic drugs periodically (Table 1).

From a non-pharmacological perspective, she was treated in the center's psychology department. Psychologists detected family problems, poor socialization, and a lack of acceptance of the disease with reactivity to support proposals, such as technical aids for ambulation or functional independence. She also attended therapeutic programs of the Spanish National Organization for the Blind (ONCE), where she currently receives supportive psychotherapy and participates in activities such as gymnastics and choir. Regarding physical activity, ONCE provides cardiorespiratory and muscular maintenance as well as psychomotor coordination training.

2.5. Supplementary Tests

The patient's multiple pathologies and her evolution have required the performance of different complementary tests, the chronology and results of which are summarized in Tables 2 and 3. In August 2019, a routine electrocardiogram (ECG) was performed, showing atrial fibrillation (AF) at 120 bpm, initiating treatment with digoxin, diltiazen, and low molecular weight heparin (LMWH). Examined by the cardiology service, an echocardiogram was performed, which showed multiple valve disease, adjusting the treatment (Table 1).

Table 2. Control serum parameters.

Parameter/Year	2014	2018	2019	2020	2021-1	2021-2
TSH	4.22	niop	4.50	4.96	2.30	2.95
T3	8.2	niop	8.7	niop	7.5	6.5
T4	0.9	niop	0.9	niop	0.8	0.8
Vit D	niop	niop	niop	34.6	42.77	39.1
Glu	112	115	125	136	156	151
Hgb A1c	6.2	6.1	niop	niop	6,6	6.1
Cholesterol	288	224	240	155	164	171
HDL	58	47	41	43	49	52
LDL	214	162	150	90	82	100
Triglicéridos	80	77	81	110	165	93
Digoxinemia	niop	niop	niop	niop	niop	0.8

Note: 2021-1 (February 2021). 2021-2 (October 2021). Parameters in mg/dl. Hgb A1c in %. Digoxinemia in nanograms/mL. niop: not included or provided.

Table 3. Control cardiac and psychological paremeters.

Parameter/Year	2014	2018	2019	2020	2021-1	2021-2
SBP	120	135	116	125	150	135
DBP	65	66	67	70	75	70
Heart rate	80	80	120	80	70	72
SO%	niop	99	niop	niop	96	96
ECG	niop	niop	AF	AF	AF	AF
Test						
GADS	-	-	-	-	8/5	7/0

Note: 2021-1 (February 2021). 2021-2 (October 2021). AF (Atrial Fiblilation). GADS: Goldberg Anxiety and Depression Scale. niop: not included or provided.

Assessed in August 2020, in neurology outpatient clinics in relation to a double episode of nocturnal disorientation, a cranial CT scan was requested that found a "small cerebellar hemorrhage" requiring hospitalization for neurological surveillance. Treatment with edobaxan is preventedly suspended due to its anticoagulant properties. A brain study is completed with MRI that does not clearly show the presence of hemorrhage, ruling out malformations or other lesions that cause bleeding. There was good evolution during the hospital stay. A control cranial CT scan was performed that showed a punctiform image in the right cerebellar hemisphere corresponding to calcification, so the patient was discharged and the edobaxan regimen was restarted.

During the COVID-19 pandemic, a SARS CoV-2 antigen screening was performed (November 2020) with a negative result.

2.6. Follow-Up during 2021

In December 2020, the patient went to the new FM service of the center showing a defective speech related to her visual difficulties, including a negativistic discourse with complaints as well as a nihilistic view of her circumstances and her future. She also maintained her heart disease, brain damage, anxiety-depressive symptoms, side effects of drug treatment, and secondary functional dependence. The clinical examination showed a temperature of 35.7 °C, heart rate of 70 bpm (atrial fibrillation), blood pressure of 150/75 mmHg, and O_2 saturation of 96%, resulting in normal physical and neurological examination. She reports complex visual hallucinations (people, animals, and objects) in the absence of cognitive impairment that appears to be Charles Bonnet syndrome.

During the months of January and June 2021, she attended four times for analytical control, assessment of the evolution and therapeutic adjustment (see Tables 1–3), in coordination with her cardiologist and her psychiatrist. Different analytical parameters have been requested including hemogram, proteinogram, kidney function tests, and glomerular filtration. Hepatopancreatic, ionogram, markers of heart failure such as NT pro-BNP, iron metabolism, and anemias screening have shown data suggestive of normality.

The SARS-COVID-19 immunization is carried out between the months of March and April 2021.

In consultation with her FM and carried out in October 2021, the patient attends in the company of her husband; she is very cooperative, smiling, and showing emotional stability, with absence of parasuicidal ideation and Charles Bonnet syndrome, which she associates with increased physical activity and psychotherapeutic as well as to correct pharmacological control, despite the fact that anxiety levels remain high, referring to fear of loss of family support (the results are shown in Tables 1–3).

3. Case Management from Family Medicine

Since it is a patient who lives in the community, the FM department of the health center has acted, coordinating the needs of monitoring of the different pathologies that she presents with the support of her family as a basic element of well-being. It is a classic FM strategy, implemented with the aim of achieving primary, secondary, and tertiary prevention.

4. Discussion

In the present case, the following areas of deliberation are raised: 1. Multifactorial etiology of the disease; 2. Diagnostic certainty; 3. Efficacy of psychopharmacological treatment; and 4. Role of the family in the patient's care.

4.1. Multifactorial Etiology of the Disease

The main risk factors for depressive disorder in old adults have been frequently studied and include psychosocial circumstances of the aging process, personality factors, previous psychiatric pathology, intercurrent illnesses, and the interactions of associated treatments, although the level of influence of each factor is difficult to discriminate [18,19].

The present case could constitute a paradigm of the multicausality of depressive disorder in old adulthood, since, in a progressive and continuous way, several of the main factors associated with depressive symptoms that contribute to chronicity have been presented. In the psychosocial level, losses and grief, loneliness, environmental changes, and maladjustment stand out as potential etiological factors [20]. In this case, she is a person with a high cultural level, economic resources, comfortable habitat, and very stable social and family support. Regarding personality factors, some authors suggest that traits such as neuroticism increase the risk of presenting depressive symptoms in old adulthood [21]. It was not considered necessary to assess personality factors in a structured way, since an evolution of 10 years and the previous therapeutic approaches seem to be advisable, although it is true that the patient frequently refers to "a change in personality, from shyness to a certain disinhibition in the last years" associated with the general clinical picture that could be the result of antidepressant treatment. In the medical history, no references to previous psychiatric pathologies, consumption of toxic substances, or adjustment disorders were observed, with a stable work environment until her retirement.

Different studies associate metabolic diseases such as hypothyroidism and diabetes mellitus, or cardio and cerebrovascular disease, with an increased risk of suffering from depression, relating it to the multiple neuroimmunoendocrine changes in depressive patients. It has been observed that patients with depressive symptoms experience increased platelet activation that could predispose them to thromboembolic episodes. They also experience immune activation (NK cells and leukocytes) and hypercortisolemia, along with an increased adrenocorticotropic hormone (ACTH) and ACTH-releasing factor. In addition, they experience decreased insulin resistance, increased endogenous production of steroids, and the release of catecholamines, associated with an increase in arterial pressure and coronary vasoconstriction. Moreover, depressive symptoms constitute a poor prognostic factor in cardiovascular and metabolic diseases [22–25]. In this case, the protocol-based examinations showed no alteration justifying the role of physical factors in the depressive simptomatology. On the other hand, the polypharmacy used to control these diseases constitutes a known precipitating factor of depressive symptoms in old adults. Thus, drugs such as digoxin, diuretics, oral antidiabetics, and antihypertensives have been frequently associated with a greater risk of depression in these populations [26]. We cannot determine the level of influence of these drugs on the prognosis, but we can consider that their interactions with antidepressant drugs could make remission of the depressive symptomatology difficult.

In the clinical evolution of the patient, we consider the loss of vision to be key in the chronification of depressive symptoms due to the psychological repercussions as a factor of anxiety, insecurity, and fear; the functional repercussions for the instrumental and basic activities of daily life that limit self-care and potentiate iatrogenic risks; and the social repercussions related to leisure activities and increased consumption of resources, all of which favor frailty and limit self-perception of health status.

On the other hand, we consider the presence of a Charles Bonnet syndrome characterized by hallucinations to be of interest, which are commonly perceived as real by the patients and are related to visual deficits. Although the underlying mechanism is not well understood, it seems to be related to a brain's continuous adjustment to significant vision loss. Old adults affected with Charlet Bonnet syndrome can avoid reporting to their doctor because of fear that the hallucinations could be related to a severe mental disorder. The clinical management consists of health education, explaining to the patient the nature of the disorder, the prevalent symptomatology, making them aware of the symptoms, and explaining that it is part of their visual deficit and not relevant to their depressive symptomatology. Eventually, pharmacological treatment with neuroleptics, benzodiazepines, antidepressants, and antiepileptics is required [16,17].

4.2. Diagnosis of Depression

As a complex diagnosis, major depression in old age involves assessing cognitive functions, behaviors, and the impact of any affective disorder on the functional capacity and quality of life of the patient. Following the DSM-5 criteria [11] facilitates the discrimination between a depressive disorder and a mixed adjustment disorder that could be better explained according to the current situation of the process. For the diagnosis of major depressive disorder, the criterion of temporality greater than two weeks, the presence of a depressed mood most of the day, and anhedonia, or a marked decrease in interest or a displeasure in almost all activities, are included; in addition, the presence of at least five additional symptoms are included, such as insomnia, hyporexia, loss of energy, inappropriate feelings of guilt and worthlessness, and self-destructive ideation, among others. In the case of mixed adjustment disorder, the diagnostic criteria include five groups (A–E), so that the anxiety-depressive symptoms occur in response to an identifiable stressor or factors that occur in the following three months. At the beginning of the stressor (A), the symptoms are clinically relevant with an intense and disproportionate discomfort in relation to the intensity of the stressor, generating a significant deterioration of social functioning or of other areas (B), other mental disorders are excluded (C), the symptoms do not represent a normal grief (D), and once the stressful event or its consequences have ended, the symptoms do not persist for more than another six months (E). In the case reported, it is not possible to fulfill criterion E because the most significant stress factors, those that generate the most discomfort and maladjustment, have become chronic so their resolution is not possible. Structured cognitive assessment has not been carried out because of the absence of progressive decline.

4.3. Efficacy of the Psychopharmacological Treatment

As has been reported, the pharmacological approach in this case is highly complex. Until the advent of SSRIs, the treatments of choice were TCA and tetracyclic (ATTC) antidepressants, but the potential induction of anticholinergic effects can cause cardiovascular alterations (orthostatic hypotension, arrhythmias, electrocardiographic alterations), changes in intestinal motility (constipation, paralytic ileus), urinary retention, and pupillary dilatation, among others, discouraging their use. Currently, SSRIs and SSNRIs are the dominant pharmacological approaches for depression in old adults, motivated by their ease of use, versatility, efficacy, and safety, in addition to their cost-effectiveness.

SSRIs (fluoxetine, fluvoxamine, paroxetine, sertraline, citalopram, escitalopram) work by blocking the reuptake of serotonin (5-HT) through inhibition of the adenosine triphosphatase (ATPase)-dependent sodium/potassium transporter (NA+/K+) in presynaptic neurons. With some differences between them, they have effects on other neurotransmission systems such as noradrenergic or dopaminergic. They are metabolized by liver enzymes, especially cytochrome P450 2D6, and have different pharmacokinetic characteristics. The main indication is major depression, although they are also useful in conditions such as obsessive-compulsive disorder or anxiety disorders. The most frequent side effects are gastrointestinal (nausea, burning, diarrhea), related to intestinal 5-HT receptors, which are minimized with a staggered dosage of medication. A variable percentage of patients treated with SSRIs manifest a sensation of activation of the central nervous system with agitation, nervousness, and insomnia that usually responds to moderate doses of benzodiazepines, such as alprazolam, lorazepam, or clonazepam. In general, they present a moderate risk of pharmacological interactions, and they are very safe drugs, as studies of lethal overdose show [27–32].

SSNRIs, such as duloxetine and venlafaxine, are a second group of drugs especially useful in the treatment of depression in old adulthood. SSNRIs may have a faster onset of action than other antidepressants by modulation of beta-adrenergic receptors. Duloxetine is a potent 5-HT and norepinephrine reuptake inhibitor with low affinity for muscarinic or histamine receptors, whereas venlafaxine shares 5-HT reuptake potency with moderate effects on norepinephrine reuptake and few effects on other neurotransmission systems. In addition, they present a low risk of pharmacokinetic interactions due to low potency in the inhibition of liver enzymes of cytochrome P450, a factor that facilitates their use. The FDA indications for this group of drugs are major depression, generalized anxiety disorder, and social anxiety disorder. Since they have a mechanism of action similar to that of tricyclic antidepressants, SSNRIs have shown their usefulness in some pain disorders, which makes them especially useful in older patients and in depression associated with neuropathic comorbidity. They share some of the gastrointestinal side effects with SSRIs, however, they differ from these in the moderate risk of increased blood pressure, somewhat less frequently in prolonged-release venlafaxine, which requires periodic monitoring in the first months of treatment and is solved by adjusting the dose. Other side effects described are syncope, ortostatic hypotension, and anticholinergic symptoms, such as dry mouth, urinary retention, and constipation, which in old patients must be monitored. Exceptional cases of fatal overdose have been described. Its level of efficacy compared to SSRIs seems somewhat higher, even though the data are discrepant [33–38].

In recent years, the approval of mirtazapine for the treatment of depression has led to its frequent use in old adults. It is an antagonist of alpha 2-adrenergic receptors that acts by increasing the release of norepinephrine that achieves a rapid increase in 5-HT levels, achieving modulation of the serotonergic system. Mirtazapine is metabolized through cytochrome P450 enzymes without being an inducer or inhibitor of these enzymes, so there are no interactions with other psychotropic agents, which facilitates the combination. Its main indication is major depression, used alone or in association with SSRIs/SSNRIs. Compared with paroxetine, it showed a faster response and fewer dropouts associated with adverse effects. Among the most frequent side effects are drowsiness (which advises its use at night) and increased appetite and weight. Furthermore, it seems to increase the levels of cholesterol and triglycerides secondarily, which, associated with its potential cardiovascular effect, makes it necessary to monitor blood pressure [39–41].

The therapeutic strategy is of great interest in this case. Since it is a highly complex case, the management of psychotropic drugs had to be careful, requiring consideration not only of the efficacy and probability of remission, but also of the minimization of secondary organic complications, to guarantee safety. In addition, the progressive appearance of comorbid, cardio, and cerebrovascular factors has required pharmacological adjustment. The potential interactions of the treatment must be considered, with the aim being its optimization. We consider the combined use of venlafaxine and mirtazapine to be successful due to its efficacy and safety, as evidenced by the adequate adherence of the patient to treatment and medical controls. In the case of duloxetine, its potential modification of blood pressure levels could question its use in this case [42]. The Goldberg Anxiety and Depression Scale (GADS) carried out in October 2021 suggests a remission of depressive symptoms and an improvement in the patient's attitude. However, based on the results of the interview and the GADS (A7/D0), the use of benzodiazepines to control anxiety and insomnia symptoms does not seem clear.

4.4. Role of the Family in the Patient's Care

This case presents many of the specific challenges in managing geriatric patients in the Galician health care model (northwest Spain). The guarantee of citizens' health rights has been defined in the Spanish constitution since 1978. However, in 2002 there was a decentralization of competences in different areas, including health, according to the Law of Cohesion and Quality of the National Health System, which established a framework in the 17 autonomous communities of the Spanish State, but with peculiarities according to each territory. Regardless of this framework, the citizens, using their freedom, choose in each health situation whether to be treated in the public health system (in Galicia, the Servicio Galego de Saúde, or SERGAS) or in the free market system (private clinical services companies and/or consultations by private professionals), or both. The reality is that this mixed system can condition the efficiency of geriatric and psychiatric interventions in complex cases, hindering actions from primary health care because decision-making is dispersed. In this context, relevant information for therapeutic optimization is frequently lost.

The socioeconomic context of the patient allows clinical follow-up with good health resources, within a dual system (private and public) that contributes to effective health care, although its efficiency is limited by the heterogeneity of clinical opinions. As it has been mentioned above, the health care model in Galicia is based on a public, universal system in coexistence with private companies and entities of the social sector that provide health and care services, in addition to freelance professionals in health areas such as ophthalmology, psychiatry, internal medicine, or psychology, among many others. Between 2020 and 2021, the COVID-19 pandemic has required the adoption of restrictive measures in terms of prevention and mobility attitudes that seem to increase the incidence of psychiatric pathology in old populations [43,44], although in this case it does not seem to have conditioned the evolution of the patient.

We believe that a more intensive non-pharmacological approach would contribute to improving the prognosis; specifically, it would reduce anxiety-type symptoms and achieve a more objective self-perception of health. It would be an area for improvement using some of the usual techniques in similar cases, from cognitive behavioral to supportive or family therapy. In recent years, third generation behavioral therapies seem to contribute to intervention in psychogeriatrics. These include Acceptance and Commitment Therapy, Dialectical Behavioral Therapy, Mindfulness-Based Therapy, Behavioral Activation Therapy, Integral Behavioral Couple Therapy, or Functional Analytical Psychotherapy, which share an integrative vision of the psychological problems of old patients, considering their functional structure relevant, that is, the psychological functions of maladaptive behaviors in the context in which they occur [45]. These types of approaches may probably contribute to improve the quality of life and the health perception of the patient.

The evolution of the depressive disorder is linked to the role that her husband plays in psychological care and functional support for her activities of daily living. The long duration of the disease and the appearance of associated pathologies increase the intensity of care. The parallel aging of the husband and the incidence of medical and psychological problems could contribute to a potential claudication or the development of caregiver burnout [46,47].

5. Conclusions

The present work discusses the complexity of the diagnosis and treatment of depression in the geriatric patient. It is illustrated with the case of a patient (a 75-year-old woman) with depressive symptomatology with more than 10 years of evolution, also affected by different concomitant organic pathologies including visual deficits and Charles Bonnet syndrome. The interventions of different medical specialties are shown, and some psychopharmacological treatment options are discussed. The interactions of the different pharmacological treatments and the mixed care approaches are considered, with the aims of improving the case management and maximizing the quality of life of the patient in this type of complex clinical condition. The complexity of the healthcare system in Galicia (northwest Spain) and how difficult it is to handle complex geriatric cases in this context are discussed. In this regard, the most relevant limitation of this case in the lack of a specific approach, substituted for this patient by a mixed care model. Other limitations include the lack of a personality assessment using psychometrically valid tests, the lack of an explicit frailty assessment beyond the clinical observation of an increased bio-psycho-social vulnerability, and the lack of an objective assessment of the caregiver burden.

Author Contributions: J.C.-P. and M.G.D. conceived and designed the case report; J.C.-P., M.G.D., M.P.P., A.d.l.I.C. and M.E.C. collected the data and prepared the case report; D.F. critically reviewed the case report and prepared contributions regarding depression disorders and psycho-social care. All authors reviewed and revised the manuscript. All authors have read and agreed to the published version of the manuscript.

Funding: This research received no external funding.

Institutional Review Board Statement: This study was conducted in accordance with the Declaration of Helsinki. As a single case report, ethical review and approval was not applicable.

Informed Consent Statement: Informed consent, following the recommendation of the Galician Clinical Research Ethics Committee, was obtained from the participant.

Data Availability Statement: The data presented in this study can be requested to the corresponding author. The data are not publicly available due to confidentiality and anonymity.

Conflicts of Interest: All authors declare no conflict of interest.

References

1. Mañana Rendal, P.M. Depresión y ansiedad. In *Gerontología y Geriatría: Valoración e intervención*; Calentí, M., Ed.; Médica Panamericana: Madrid, Spain, 2010; pp. 285–301.
2. Blazer, D.G. Depression in Late Life: Review and Commentary. *J. Gerontol. A Biol. Sci. Med. Sci* **2003**, *58*, 249–265. [CrossRef]
3. Diego Calderón, M. Epidemiología de la depresión en el adulto mayor. *Rev. Med. Hered.* **2018**, *29*, 182–191. [CrossRef]
4. Sotelo-Alonso, I.; Rojas-Soto, J.E.; Sánchez-Arenas, C.; Irigoyen-Coria, A. Depresión en el adulto mayor: Una perspectiva clínica y epidemiológica desde el primer nivel de atención. *Arch. Med. Fam.* **2012**, *14*, 5–13.
5. Pando Moreno, M.; Aranda Beltrán, C.; Alfaro Alfaro, N.; Mendoza Roaf, P. Prevalencia de depresión en adultos mayores en población urbana. *Rev. Esp. Geriatr. Gerontol.* **2001**, *36*, 140–144. [CrossRef]
6. Anton Jiménez, M.; Gálvez Sánchez, N.; Esteban Saiz, R. *Tratado de Geriatría para Residentes. Depresión y Ansiedad*; Sociedad Española de Geriatría y Gerontología: Madrid, Spain, 2006.
7. Zarebski, G. Factores de riesgo psíquico de envejecimiento patológico y factores protectores. In *Cuestionario Mi Envejecer. Un Instrumento Psicogerontológico para Evaluar la Actitud Frente al Propio Envejecimiento*; En Zarebski, G., Ed.; Paidós: Buenos Aires, Argentina, 2014; pp. 37–50.
8. Biermann, T.; Sperling, W.; Bleich, S.; Kornhuber, J.; Reulbach, H. Particularities of suicide in the elderly. A population-based study. *Aging Clin. Exp. Res.* **2009**, *21*, 470–474. [CrossRef]
9. Ferraris, L.; Lopez, G. Depresión y envejecimiento: Complejidades del diagnóstico y abordaje (Caso clínico). *Neurama Revista Electrónica de Psicogeriatría* **2017**, *4*, 45–49.
10. World Health Organization. *ICD-10 Classification of Mental and Behavioural Disorders: Clinical Descriptions and Diagnostic Guidelines*; World Health Organization: Geneva, Switzerland, 1992.
11. American Psychiatric Association. *Diagnostic and Statistical Manual of Mental Disorders (DSM–5)*; American Psychiatric Association: Philadelphia, PA, USA, 2013.
12. Gil Gregorio, P.; Martín Carrasco, M. *Guía de Buena Práctica Clínica en Geriatría. Depresión y Ansiedad*; Sociedad Española de Geriatría y Gerontología: Madrid, Spain, 2004.
13. Frank, C. Pharmacologic treatment of depression in the elderly. *Can. Fam. Physician* **2014**, *60*, 121–126.
14. Alexopoulos, G.S. Pharmacotherapy for late-life depression. *J. Clin. Psychiatry* **2011**, *72*, e04. [CrossRef]
15. Balo García, A.; González-Abraldes, I. Intervención no Farmacológica y con Cuidadores. In *Gerontología y Geriatría: Valoración e intervención*; Calentí, M., Ed.; Médica Panamericana: Madrid, Spain, 2010; pp. 303–319.
16. Jan, T.; del Castillo, J. Visual hallucinations: Charles BonnetsSyndrome. *West. J. EmergMed.* **2012**, *13*, 544–547. [CrossRef]
17. García Fraga, J.A.; López Rego, L.; Mayán Cones, P.; Serrano Vázquez, M. Síndrome de Charles Bonnet. *Rev. Esp. Geriatr. Gerontol.* **2007**, *42*, 60–61. [CrossRef]
18. Beekman, A.T.; de Beurs, E.; van Balkom, A.J.; Deeg, D.J.; van Dyck, R.; van Tilburg, W. Anxiety and depression in later life: Co-occurrence and communality of risk factors. *Am. J. Psychiatry* **2000**, *157*, 89–95. [CrossRef] [PubMed]
19. Vilalta-Franch, J.; Planas-Pujol, X.; Lopez-Pousa, S.; Llinas-Regla, J.; Merino-Aguado, J.; Garre-Olmo, J. Depression subtypes and 5-years risk of mortality in aged 70 years: A population-based cohort study. *Int. J. Geriatr. Psychiatry* **2011**, *27*, 67–75. [CrossRef] [PubMed]
20. Sözeri-Varma, G. Depression in the elderly: Clinical features and risk factors. *Aging Dis.* **2012**, *3*, 465–471. [PubMed]
21. Hayward, R.D.; Taylor, W.D.; Smoski, M.J.; Steffens, D.C.; Payne, M.E. Association of NEO personality domains and facets with presence, onset, and treatment outcomes of major depression in older adults. *Am. J. Geriatr. Psychiatry* **2013**, *21*, 88–96. [CrossRef]
22. Pintor, L. Insuficiencia cardiaca y enfermedad depresiva, una frecuente combinación tantas veces olvidada. *Rev. Esp. Cardiol.* **2006**, *59*, 761–765. [CrossRef]
23. Lett, H.S.; Blumenthal, J.A.; Babyak, M.A.; Sherwood, A.; Strauman, T.; Robins, C.; Newman, M.F. Depression as a risk factor for coronary artery disease: Evidence, mechanisms, and treatment. *Psychosom. Med.* **2004**, *66*, 305–315.
24. Turvey, C.L.; Klein, D.M.; Pies, C.J. Depression, physical impairment, and treatment of depression in chronic heart failure. *J. Cardiovasc. Nurs.* **2006**, *21*, 175–178. [CrossRef]
25. López, S.; Gasull, V.; Alcalá, J.A. *Depresión mayor: Recomendaciones SEMERGEN*; Editorial Medical & Marketing Comunications: Madrid, Spain, 2016; pp. 8–38.
26. Alcalde, P.; Dapena, M.D.; Nieto, M.D.; Fontecha, B.J. Ingreso hospitalario atribuible a efectos adversos a medicamentos. *Rev. Esp. Geriatr. Gerontol.* **2001**, *36*, 340–344. [CrossRef]
27. Schatzberg, A.F.; Cole, J.O.; DeBattista, C. *Manual of Clinical Psychopharmacology*; American Psychiatric Association: Washington, DC, USA, 2003.
28. Schatzberg, A.F.; Nemeroff, C.B. *Textbook of Psychopharmacology*, 5th ed.; American Psychiatric Association: Washington, DC, USA, 2017.

29. Cole, M.G.; Elie, L.M.; McCusker, J.; Bellavance, F.; Mansour, A. Feasibility and effectiveness of treatments for depression in elderly medical inpatients: A systematic review. *Int. Psychogeriatr.* **2000**, *12*, 453–461. [CrossRef]
30. Magni, L.R.; Purgato, M.; Gastaldon, C.; Papola, D.; Furukawa, T.A.; Cipriani, A.; Barbui, C. Fluoxetine versus other types of pharmacotherapy for depression. *Cochrane Database Syst. Rev.* **2013**, *17*, CD004185. [CrossRef]
31. Purgato, M.; Papola, D.; Gastaldon, C.; Trespidi, C.; Magni, L.R.; Rizzo, C.; Furukawa, T.A.; Watanabe, N.; Cipriani, A.; Barbui, C. Paroxetine versus other anti-depressive agents for depression. *Cochrane Database Syst. Rev.* **2014**, *3*, CD006531. [CrossRef]
32. Muñiz-Schwochert, R.; Olazarán-Rodríguez, J.; López-Álvarez, J.; Agüera-Ortiz, L.F.; López-Arrieta, J.M.; Beltrán-Aguirre, J.L.; García-García, P.; Rigueira-García, A.; Martín-Carrasco, M.; Qintana-Hernández, D.J. Criterios CHROME para la acreditación de centros libres de sujeciones químicas y para una prescripción de psicofármacos de calidad. *Psicogeriatría* **2016**, *6*, 91–98.
33. Norris, S.; Blier, P. Duloxetine, milnacipram and levomilnacipram. In *Textbook of Psychopharmacology*, 5th ed.; American Psychiatric Association: Washington, DC, USA, 2017; pp. 529–548.
34. Wise, T.N.; Wiltse, C.G.; Iosifescu, D.V.; Sheridan, M.; Xu, J.I.; Raskin, J. The safety and tolerability of duloxetine in depressed elderly patients with and without medical comorbidity. *Int. J. Clin. Pract.* **2007**, *61*, 1283–1293. [CrossRef] [PubMed]
35. Raskin, J.; Xu, J.Y.; Kajdasz, D.K. Time to response for duloxetine 60 mg once daily versus placebo in elderly patients with major depressive disorder. *Int. Psychogeriatr.* **2008**, *20*, 309–327. [CrossRef] [PubMed]
36. Thase, M.E. Venlafaxine and desvenlafaxine. In *Textbook of Psychopharmacology*, 5th ed.; American Psychiatric Association: Washington, DC, USA, 2017.
37. Kirby, D.; Harrigan, S.; Ames, D. Hyponatraemia in elderly psychiatric patients treated with Selective Serotonin Reuptake Inhibitors and venlafaxine: A retrospective controlled study in an inpatient unit. *Int. J. Geriatr. Psychiatry* **2002**, *17*, 231–237. [CrossRef] [PubMed]
38. Dyer, A.H.; Murphy, C.; Briggs, R.; Lawlor, B.; Kennelly, S.P.; NILVAD Study Group. Antidepressant use and orthostatic hypotension in older adults living with mild-to-moderate Alzheimer disease. *Int. J. Geriatr. Psychiatry* **2020**, *35*, 1367–1375. [CrossRef] [PubMed]
39. Schatzberg, A.F. Mirtazapine. In *Textbook of Psychopharmacology*, 5th ed.; American Psychiatric Association: Washington, DC, USA, 2017.
40. Schatzberg, A.F.; Kremer, C.; Rodrigues, H.E.; Murphy, G.M., Jr. Double-blind, randomized comparison of mirtazapine and paroxetine in elderly depressed patients. *Am. J. Geriatr. Psychiatry* **2002**, *10*, 541–550. [CrossRef] [PubMed]
41. Behlke, L.M.; Lenze, E.J.; Carney, R.M. The cardiovascular effects of newer antidepressants in older adults and those with or at high risk for cardiovascular diseases. *CNS Drugs* **2020**, *34*, 1133–1147. [CrossRef]
42. Hannan, N.; Hamzah, Z.; Akinpeloye, H.O.; Meagher, D. Venlafaxine-mirtazapine combination in the treatment of persistent depressive illness. *J. Psychopharmacol.* **2007**, *21*, 161–164. [CrossRef] [PubMed]
43. Picaza Gorrochategi, M.; Eiguren Munitis, A.E.; Dosil Santamaria, M.; Ozamiz Etxebarria, N. Stress, anxiety, and depression in people aged over 60 in the COVID-19 outbreak in a sample collected in northern Spain. *Am. J. Geriatr. Psychiatry* **2020**, *28*, 993–998. [CrossRef]
44. Aranda Rubio, Y.; Aranda Rubio, L.; Alcaraz-L, C.; Isach Comallonga, M. Repercusiones en la salud mental del paciente anciano tras padecer COVID-19: Trastorno de estrés postraumático. A propósito de un caso. *Rev. Esp. Geriatr. Gerontol.* **2021**, *56*, 115–116. [CrossRef]
45. Márquez-González, M. Nuevas herramientas para la intervención psicológica con personas mayores: La tercera generación de terapias conductuales. *Rev. Esp. Geriatr. Gerontol.* **2021**, *45*, 247–249. [CrossRef] [PubMed]
46. Pérez-Salanova, M.; Yanguas-Lezaun, J.J. Dependencia, personas mayores y familias. De los enunciados a las intervenciones. *An. Psicol.* **1998**, *14*, 95–104.
47. Acker, G.M.; Lawrence, D. Social work and managed care: Measuring competence, burnout, and role stress of workers providing mental health services in a managed care era. *J. Soc. Work* **2009**, *9*, 269–283. [CrossRef]

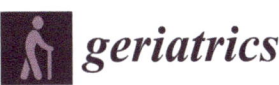

Case Report

Behavioral Interventions in Long-Term Care Facilities during the COVID-19 Pandemic: A Case Study

Carlos Dosil-Díaz [1,2,*], David Facal [2] and Romina Mouriz-Corbelle [1,2]

1. Gerontological Therapeutic Complex "A Veiga", Serge Lucense, Pobra de San Xiao, 27360 Lancara, Spain; romina.mouriz@usc.es
2. Department of Developmental Psychology, University of Santiago de Compostela, 15782 Santiago de Compostela, Spain; david.facal@usc.es
* Correspondence: carlos.dosil@usc.es; Tel.: +34-670861981

Abstract: During the COVID-19 pandemic, long-term care (LTC) centers have adopted a series of measures that have affected the physical and cognitive health of patients. The routines of the patients, as well as the interventions of professionals, have been altered. In the case presented here, our aim was to explain the effect that the strong confinement due to the spread of the first COVID-19 wave in Spain had on a 75-year-old resident in an LTC center, with cognitive and behavioral symptomatology compatible with a diagnosis of mixed dementia, as well as the measures that the center adopted to manage the lockdown situation in the best possible way, including personalized attention protocols and a video call program. Different nosological hypotheses are also raised using a semiological analysis, including the analysis of the initial and continuation diagnostic protocols, as well as the therapeutic options.

Keywords: mixed dementia; behavioral and psychological symptoms in dementia; challenging behaviors; lockdown

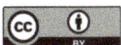

1. Introduction

In March 2020, long-term care (LTC) centers were dramatically affected in their operations by the COVID-19 pandemic. The high rate of frailty of the old residents caused a disproportionate number of deaths during the first wave of the pandemic, reaching 20% in centers that were affected by COVID-19. The centers implemented a series of measures to deal with COVID-19, including the sectorization of spaces, use of PPE, controls of daily constants, reorganization of functions in the staff, and the restriction or elimination of visits from relatives to residents, among others [1]. Different studies show that the pandemic has had a very negative impact on institutionalized older people and, more specifically, on those who suffer cognitive impairment with behavioral alterations, due, to a large extent, to the fact that the restrictions on social relationships increase the problems of loneliness and isolation, which existed before the pandemic [2].

In LTC centers, 60–80% of patients have some degree of cognitive impairment, 20–30% show severe phase dementia, and 65% have some behavioral disorder [3]. In this way, patients suffering from dementia, in addition to presenting an important alteration in cognitive functions, due to the progressive deterioration of some brain functions, show the Behavioral and Psychological Symptoms of Dementia (BPSD). It has been described that between 60% and 90% of patients with dementia will present BPSD throughout the course of the disease [4]. This percentage varies depending on the stage and the previous personality of the patient. Behavioral symptoms refer to physical aggression, yelling, restlessness, wandering, culturally inappropriate behaviors, sexual disinhibition, harassment, inappropriate language, and persistent following of another. Psychological symptoms refer to anxiety problems, depressed mood, hallucinations and delusions, etc. [5]. One of the models used to address the management of behavior disorders is that of Cohen-Mansfield [6]. In this model, the needs of the person with dementia and professionals caring for them are considered, as well as clinical and environmental characteristics. The intervention, therefore, arises from a paradigm of personalized care, where the person is the center of the intervention, and the professional must adapt to the patient's needs.

In this sense, it is important to highlight that LTC center residents often present disruptive symptoms, which increases the stress of the caregivers and the suffering of the person with dementia, sometimes reaching the need to use physical restraints and/or drugs to alleviate these symptoms [7]. For all these reasons, it is essential to carry out an interdisciplinary intervention focused on older residents. Although the tendency is to increase this type of tailorized interventions in LTC centers, during the COVID-19 pandemic, this has been hampered by the measures taken to contain the spread of the virus [8]. The present manuscript is a case study that addresses the intervention of a patient admitted to a residential LTC center during the first wave of the COVID-19 pandemic.

2. Materials and Methods

2.1. Case

2.1.1. Personal History

The resident is 75 years old, a woman, and a widow, and she has three children. She was born in the rural area of Sarria, Lugo (Galicia, Spain). She entered the LTC center in January 2020. Until admission, she lived alone. She was a very active woman and ran a store for decades and she had a basic education.

2.1.2. Medical and Psychological History

The resident presented dementia with a mixed profile and behavioral alterations, hypertensive heart disease, permanent atrial fibrillation, dyslipidemia, and osteoporosis. The information provided came from the reports of the relatives, as well as the social reports of the town hall and the clinical reports of the hospital.

In June 2018, a cranial CT scan was performed without intravenous contrast, showing no evidence of space-occupying lesions in an intraparenchymal or extra-axial location. There was supratentorial predominance of white matter, in periventricular and subcritical locations, which could correspond to leukopathy due to small vessel involvement. A revision was scheduled in September 2018 with analytical and EEG.

In August 2018, she was seen again by the specialist doctor, presenting the following symptoms: aggressiveness with the caregiver, shadowing, she had stopped cooking at home, and she was unable to perform simple memory tasks. The following treatment was prescribed: Bisprorol 2.5 mg, Digoxin 0.25, Atorvastatin 40 mg 0-0-1, Seguril 40 mg 1-0-0, Eliquis 5 mg 1-0-1, Deltius 25 mg, Rivastigmine 4.6 mg Doxium 2-0-0, and Irbesartan 300 mg 1-0-0.

In the psychological evaluation, she presented 6 errors in the Pfeiffer test, a MEC (a Spanish version of the Mini-Mental State Examination with a total score of 35) score of 21/35, and a Global Deterioration Scale (GDS) score of 4, scores that reflect moderate cognitive impairment.

In December 2018, the patient went to the hospital emergency department because she had had several syncope and falls at her home, with loss of consciousness.

During the year 2019, she stayed at her home supervised by her children, and in January 2020, she entered the A Veiga Xerontolóxico Therapeutic Complex, three months before the COVID-19 pandemic was declared in Spain.

2.1.3. Status When Entering the LTC Center

Upon arrival, she was evaluated by the LTC center doctor in coordination with the referral geriatrician at the Lucus Augusti hospital. They observed that she presented flight delirium, anosognosia due to cognitive impairment, and independence in BADL without execution errors. Behavioral alterations stood out, with poor management with current treatment. An ECG was performed to rule out repolarization alterations in the face of blockages.

An adjustment of the medication was made taking into account the rejection that the patient presents to oral medicines. Seven drugs were maintained by eliminating Doxium and Irbesartan and adding two antipsychotics, Quetiapine, and a class of medication called NMDA receptor antagonists, Memantine.

In order for the psychological aspects to be evaluated, different cognitive screening tests were applied at the time of admission, including the MEC (a Spanish version of the Mini-Mental State Examination with a total score of 35), Global Deterioration Scale (GDS), and Clinical Dementia Rating (CDR) (Table 1), indicating that the resident is a person with severe cognitive impairment that includes impairment of memory, severe short-term memory circuit problems, severe temporal disorientation, and very basic spatial location, with impaired judgment, impaired problem solving, and impaired attention to personal care.

Table 1. Results of the MEC, GDS, Barthel, Yesavage, and CDR tests, applied on 31 January 2020.

Test
MEC:14
GDS: 5
Barthel Index: 85
Yesavage: 0
CDR: 2

The patient preserved communicative and relational intentionality, compensating for certain cognitive deficits. She also preserved social verbal interaction. There were reports of unfinished sentences, occasional confusion of pronunciation patterns, and difficulty naming tasks. The content of her speech included fables and misinterpretation.

The Geriatric Assessment Scale (also called Yesavage scale) was used to assess mood, obtaining an inconclusive result (Table 1) given the unreliability of the responses given by the resident.

Regarding the physiotherapeutic evaluation, the resident maintained an independent and stable gait, without the need for support products. She presented good joint balance, without stiffness and maintaining functionality. She did not present alterations in muscle tone and had a perfect general muscular balance (Daniels 5/5). In terms of balance and gait, she had a Tinetti score of 16 in balance and 12 in running, which is a low-risk assessment. Regarding the risk of falls, in the up and go test, she presented a normal risk.

To assess the functionality of the patient, we applied the Barthel Index at the time of admission. Its result indicates a moderate dependence for BADL (Table 1), such as food, transfers, personal hygiene, use of the bathroom, personal hygiene, shower, mobility, going up or down stairs, and dressing and undressing.

Taking into account the above, the different departments of the center proposed the following objectives: maintain her level of independence in the performance of the ABVD; promote her communication and relationship with other residents; encourage her participation in activities; promote her adherence to routines and guidelines; maintain her motor, cognitive, and sensory performance skills that promote functional independence; promote cognitive stimulation activities; improve her temporal and spatial orientation; etc.

In order for the set objectives to be achieved, the patient was placed in a single room on the floor intended for patients with moderate dependence (called the Red Floor) whose routines were developed on the main floor of the center, giving them the possibility of accessing different activities.

2.2. Intervention during the Lockdown

In March 2020, with the arrival of COVID-19 in Spain and the state of alarm decreed by the government of Spain, the center was divided into three large areas, which prevented normal walking through it and interaction among residents, generating an increase in their behavioral disorders, such as agitation, disinhibition, repeated calls and questions, difficulty in cleaning and manifestation of a difficult temperament, mood alterations, demanding behaviors, and apathetic behaviors with a tendency for immobility [9].

Measures derived from the COVID-19 pandemic included the confinement of residents in their bedrooms or in restricted places close to their rooms, without contact with other residents and restricted contact with their professional caregivers. Accordingly, it was necessary to rethink activities in order to achieve the achieve the therapeutical aims. Below, we expose the activities in detail:

- Attention was placed on the patient's routines, with continuous follow-up and greater support for her BADL.
- Due to the restrictions in the visitation regime (group activities and visits were suspended, according to the Decree of 17 March 2020, of the Xunta de Galicia), and since she was a person who socialized to a high degree with the residents and who had a high frequency of family visits, she was included in the center's video call program, wherein the resident could interact with her family, thus stimulating social interaction (see Figure 1).
- Personal care was also promoted, referring to hygiene, food, and clothing, as well as activities related to anti-COVID-19 measures (wearing a mask, hand disinfection). Pictograms and posters were used to facilitate these activities, wherein they were identified in a very simple way, for example, the room number with a photo of her face, posters on how to put on the mask and how to disinfect the hands, etc.

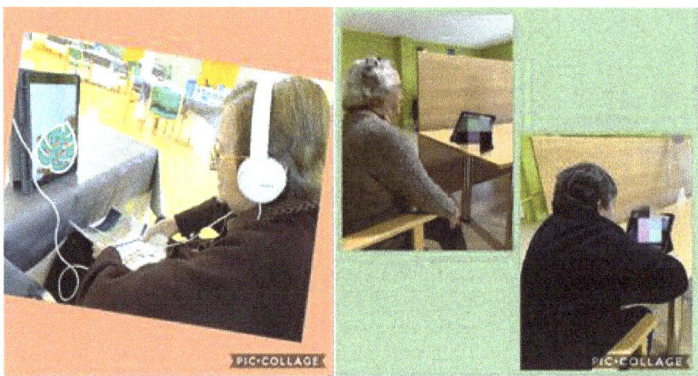

Figure 1. Video call program.

It should be noted that the patient, despite being in a sectorized area and of relative control, had serious difficulties staying in her area, mainly motivated by the cognitive impairment that she presented, with highly frequent ambulation and continuous attempts to establish contact with residents in her area and other areas.

In the last months of 2020 and early 2021, the patient experienced a worsening in BPSD (aggressiveness at bath time and personal hygiene, attempts to attack other residents, etc.). In order to guarantee adequate care for her, in March 2021, she was transferred to the psychogeriatric unit of the LTC center, which offers more specialized care that guarantees greater control, security, and supervision both for the patient herself and for the people with whom she had direct contact. In this unit, the monitoring by the medical, psychological, therapeutic, and care personnel is more intense and exhaustive. This unit has large areas, with wide corridors that favor walking. It also has a warm and homely design, with colors in light tones that help to maintain the tranquility of the residents, as well as relaxing background music. In the same way, the unit presents natural lighting, which provides a more pleasant stay. Despite being a unit where residents have high deterioration, it is about maintaining the functions and enhancing the autonomy of the residents.

Regarding the training of the personnel of the psychogeriatric unit, it should be noted that the staff have specific training that allows them to offer adequate care, emphasizing direct intervention, active roles, and feedback, despite having to work during the pandemic with a mask and protective screens. In this sense, the workers addressed the patient in a respectful way, understanding her pathology and enhancing her autonomy. The care staff of the unit were permanent personnel and that they only worked in that unit.

From the occupational therapy department, it was decided to include the resident in all the activities carried out in the psychogeriatric unit. Regarding different BPSD registered in relation to aggressiveness in grooming and dressing, aggressiveness towards other residents, and refusal to take medication, an intervention was carried out from the medical and psychological departments focused on the administration of crushed and camouflaged medication with meals, monitoring the correct intake by the medical and nursing department. Additionally, they intervened in facilitating access to her seasonal garments, removing non-corresponding garments from her wardrobe (it must be clarified that the clothes have a meaning in the patient's life history, i.e., her work occupation, as a clerk in her own clothing store). To work on her spatio-temporal orientation, a system was implemented where the patient had visual access to different objects such as clocks, paintings, and TVs, which facilitated her orientation. The form of intervention was readjusted in order to work on the aspect of functional independence to the characteristics of the unit, since it has large areas for safe ambulation as well as rest areas. For this reason, she was included in the program of walks to promote her functional independence and the redirection of excess activity.

3. Results

From the applications of different tests in three different time periods (from January 2020 to August 2021), we found a worsening of cognitive impairment in the last assessment. There was also a worsening of the BADL, measured with the Barthel Index. The other parameters remained stable (Table 2).

Table 2. Follow-up in the results of the MEC, GDS, Barthel, Yesavage, and CDR tests.

31 January 2020	30 April 2020	30 July 2021
Test	Test	Test
MEC: 14	MEC: 14	MEC: 10
GDS: 5	GDS: 5	GDS: 6
Barthel: 85	Barthel: 85	Barthel: 80
Yesavage: 0	Yesavage: 0	Yesavage: 0
CDR: 2	CDR: 2	CDR: 2

Regarding the results of the observation carried out by the staff of the unit, it was found that the most relevant problems that the patient presented were sleep disturbance and nocturnal ambulation, and, to a lesser extent, reluctance to take medication, aggressiveness during grooming and dressing, and attempted assaults on other residents. We also observed that aggressive behaviors occurred, to a large extent, when taking medication. For this reason, starting in June 2021, crushed and camouflaged medication was prescribed with meals, with the appropriate monitoring carried out. In the following months, a reduction in BPSD was observed (Table 3).

Finally, decreased agitation and improved spatio-temporal orientation; levels of attention; and, to a lesser degree, apathy were observed.

Table 3. Incidents from July 2020 to August 2021.

	Sleep Disturbance and Nocturnal Ambulation	Poor Intake and Refusal to Take Medication	Aggression at Bath Time and Personal Hygiene	Attempts to Attack Other Residents
From July to October 2020	21 incidents	1 incident	0 incident	1 incident
From November 2020 to February 2021	27 incidents	5 incident	6 incident	2 incident
From March to May 2021	19 incidents	6 incident	9 incident	0 incident
From June to August 2021	2 incidents	0 incident	0 incident	0 incident

4. Discussion

LTC centers have faced multiples challenges during the COVID-19 pandemic, including the higher risk and higher burden of the residents with BPSD [1,10–12]. Persons with BPSD present higher risks of severe COVID-19 infection due to the relation between frailty and dementia, a higher risk of severe neuropsychiatric symptoms related to delirium and encephalopathy, higher difficulty participating in screening tests, lower ability to report symptoms of infections, and higher difficulty adhering to infection control measures due to their difficulties in comprehension and remembering, and they may place themselves at higher risk of infection because of their lower abilities to maintain social isolation, to stay in one place, or to wear face masks [11]. Due to the deep impact of COVID-19 on the healthcare system, BPSD were not addressed as needed [12]. Cancellation of therapeutic activities, routine disruption, and suspension of visits and social activities have been especially challenging for these residents, forcing them to live in a stressful environment that does not fulfill their psychosocial needs [11,12]. Complementary methods to prevent BPSD consequences in the context of the COVID-19 pandemic have included direct feedback and coaching, modeling, discussions in small groups, and informative sheets providing basic information about the residents for the staff members [12]. The technology was also integrated in the interventions, although low digital competences can be an obstacle for this kind of resource [12,13]. In their study, Danilovich et al. found that a pre-existing culture of teamwork and flexibility to adopt new approaches facilitated the response to COVID-19 in LTC facilities, whereas low levels of digital literacy and low job satisfaction due to lack of face-to-face interactions hampered adaptation to the pandemic.

In the case reported, when the resident was admitted to the LTC center, she presented BPSD, as well as severe cognitive impairment measured with the MEC (score 14), which determines advanced dementia, and a moderate to severe cognitive defect, measured with the GDS (score 5). She also presented memory impairment, difficulty in retaining recent information, attention deficit, severe temporal disorientation, and very basic spatial awareness, with impaired judgment and problem solving, and moderate dependence for BADL. The resident did not manifest awareness of deterioration and/or illness.

Taking into account the results of research on the repercussions of social isolation derived from the COVID-19 pandemic, in terms of its impact on mental health both in the general population [10] and in the older adults admitted to LTC centers [2], strategies were designed aimed at slowing down, as much as possible, the advancement of dementia in the lockdown situation, especially with regard to BPSD [9]. In addition, considering that functionality worsens in dementia if adequate stimulation is not performed, the medical and psycho-social staff of the LTC center considered it ideal for this resident to follow a personalized attention program [6].

It should be noted that despite the strict measures experienced in Spanish LTC centers during in the first wave of the COVID-19 pandemic, no worsening was observed in the case study resident, even in the 4 months following the end of the lockdown. The explanation for these results is based on individualized attention and stimulation; the patient's low awareness of reality; social support during the confinement phase (video call program); and freedom in mobility through the assigned area, which allowed her brief interactions with other residents, as well as other activities already exposed, which acted as protectors of mental health and functionality. We could affirm that ICTs, through the video call program, were a very relevant social resource for the resident in that phase [2].

In the last months of 2020 and early 2021, the patient suffered a worsening of BPSD (aggressiveness at bath time and personal hygiene, attempts to attack other residents, etc.), symptoms that could be attributable, on the one hand, to the worsening of dementia, and, on the other, to the limitation of space to wander. We can say that because she always wandered through the same spaces, after a while, those distances were not enough, and therefore the resident tried to occupy private spaces or her access to certain spaces was denied/limited by preventive anti-COVID-19 measures. After an assessment of this situation by the medical and psycho-social team, in March 2021, it was decided to relocate the patient to the psychogeriatric unit, where more specialized care was offered. However, the results of the last follow-up carried out on the resident (July 2021) indicate a worsening in the cognitive and functional scores and in the basic activities of daily life.

5. Conclusions

The numerous challenges of the management of BPSD in the context of the COVID-19 pandemic have stressed the relevance of multidisciplinary, teamwork-based, and comprehensive approaches [12,13]. Measures such as the sectorization of the center, the limitation of spaces, the performance of relatively invasive tests such as taking PCR samples or antigens, the continued use of individual protection equipment, the absence of social contact, and the alteration of daily routines caused by COVID-19 predictably favored the deterioration of residents, including an increase in BPSD. In the case study described here, during the stay of the patient in the psychogeriatric unit, a series of strategies were implemented in order to minimize the effects of social isolation. In terms of promoting the resident's social contact with reference persons, ICTs were the most relevant social resource. The measures implemented helped reduce, but did not eliminate, cognitive and behavioral deterioration in the patient.

Author Contributions: Conceptualization, C.D.-D. and D.F.; methodology, C.D.-D. and D.F.; validation, C.D.-D and R.M.-C.; formal analysis, C.D.-D. and R.M.-C.; investigation, C.D.-D. and R.M.-C.; data curation, C.D.-D. and R.M.-C.; writing—original draft preparation, C.D.-D.; writing—review and editing, D.F. and R.M.-C. All authors have read and agreed to the published version of the manuscript.

Funding: This research received no external funding.

Institutional Review Board Statement: Not applicable.

Informed Consent Statement: Not applicable.

Data Availability Statement: All data will be made available upon reasonable request.

Conflicts of Interest: The authors declare that they have no conflict of interest.

References

1. American Geriatrics Society. American Geriatrics Society Policy Brief: COVID-19 and Nursing Homes. *J. Am. Geriatr. Soc.* **2020**, *68*, 908–911. [CrossRef] [PubMed]
2. Pereiro, A.X.; Dosil-Díaz, C.; Mouriz-Corbelle, R.; Pereira-Rodríguez, S.; Nieto-Vieites, A.; Pinazo-Hernandis, S.; Pinazo-Clapés, C.; Facal, D. Impact of the COVID-19 Lockdown on a Long-Term Care Facility: The Role of Social Contact. *Brain Sci.* **2021**, *11*, 986. [CrossRef] [PubMed]
3. Dosil, C.; Juncos-Rabadán, O.; Mouriz, R.; Facal, D. Sociodemographic, cognitive and health profile of people who enter residential centers in the provinces of A Coruña and Lugo. *Rev. Psicogeriatría* **2017**, *7*, 75–80.
4. Mouriz, R.; Caamaño, J.; Dosil, C.; Picón, E.; Facal, D. Apathy and agitation in institutionalized older adults, an empirically derived classification. *Psychogeriatrics* **2021**, *21*, 272–278. [CrossRef] [PubMed]
5. Azón Belarre, J.C.; Pellicer García, B.; Juárez Vela, R.; Azón Belarre, S.; Berges Usán, P.; Granada López, J.M. Prevalence of patients with psychological and behavioral symptoms of dementia and their treatment with antipsychotics. *Pilot Study North Ment. Health* **2016**, *14*, 1–19.
6. Cohen-Mansfield, J. Temporal Patterns of Agitation in Dementia. *Am. J. Geriatr. Psychiatry* **2007**, *15*, 395–405. [CrossRef]
7. Pinazo, C.; Pinazo, S.; Sales, A. Effects of an Educational Program for Professional Caregivers on Behavioral Alterations in Nursing Home Residents: Pilot Study. *J. Environ. Res. Public Health* **2020**, *17*, 8845. [CrossRef] [PubMed]

8. Livingston, G.; Weidner, W. *COVID-19 and Dementia: Difficult Decisions about Hospital Admission and Triage*; Alzheimer´s Disease International: London, UK, 2020.
9. Facal, D.; Mouriz, R.; Caamaño, J.; Dosil, C. Estrategia de abordaje de los comportamientos exigentes "challenging behaviors" en centros gerontológicos. *Conoc. Poder* **2018**, *5*, 5–12.
10. Ramírez-Ortiz, J.; Castro-Quintero, D.; Lerma-Córdoba, C.; Yela-Ceballos, F.; Escobar-Córdoba, F. Consequences of the COVID 19 pandemic on mental health associated with social isolation. *Colomb. J. Anesthesiol.* **2020**, *48*, e930. [CrossRef]
11. Keng, A.; Borwn, E.E.; Rostas, A.; Rajji, T.K.; Pollock, B.G. Effectively caring for individuals with behavioral and psychological symptoms of dementia during the COVID-19 pandemic. *Front. Psychiatry* **2020**, *11*, 573367. [CrossRef] [PubMed]
12. Debas, K.; Beauchamp, J.; Ouellet, C. Towards optimal management of behavioral and psychological symptoms of dementia: Insights from a COVID-19 pandemic experience. *Front. Psychiatry* **2021**, *12*, 634398. [CrossRef] [PubMed]
13. Danilovich, M.; Norrick, C.; Lessem, R.; Milstein, L.; Briggs, N.; Berman, R. Responding to COVID-19: Lessons learned from a senior living and social service organization. *Geriatrics* **2020**, *5*, 98. [CrossRef] [PubMed]

MDPI
St. Alban-Anlage 66
4052 Basel
Switzerland
Tel. +41 61 683 77 34
Fax +41 61 302 89 18
www.mdpi.com

Geriatrics Editorial Office
E-mail: geriatrics@mdpi.com
www.mdpi.com/journal/geriatrics

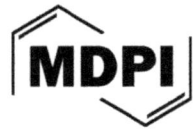

www.ingramcontent.com/pod-product-compliance
Lightning Source LLC
LaVergne TN
LVHW070045120526
838202LV00101B/469